EASY ON THE EYES

... a fresh look at vision

by Joy Thompson

Produced by:

FriesenPress

Suite 300 – 852 Fort Street
Victoria, BC, Canada V8W 1H8

www.friesenpress.com

Distributed to the trade by The Ingram Book Company

TABLE OF CONTENTS

"Speak your mind even if you are a minority of one. The truth is the truth."
— Mahatma Gandhi

PREFACE

Ever since the profoundly life-changing experience of improving my own vision and leaving my glasses on the shelf, I've wanted to inspire other people to grant themselves the same gift of restored, natural eyesight.

Could it be that in the long run, corrective prescription eyeglasses are not "corrective" at all? Could it be that glasses are a large portion of the reason why people's vision becomes weaker and weaker over the years?

Our eyes are meant to see well. Period. Just as our legs and arms and brain and lungs are designed for life-long use ... but are precious commodities, and need to be treated accordingly.

Anyone who is interested in complete health knows that eyes and eyesight must be included. Placing lenses over our eyes to help us to see in the far distance or at very close range, now and then, could be a clever way to use a tool that aids us. However, wearing prescription lenses or contacts all day, every day — or participating in elective and invasive eye surgeries — is simply not the healthy way to deal with weakened eyesight.

I'm an educator who asked a lot of questions about eyesight, and subsequently improved my vision. I went on to gain all the education I could on the subject of improving vision by natural means, and I slowly began to teach what I knew to others. What has kept me passionate all these years is the results that I see — and that my clients literally see.

Many people who put prescription lenses on in the morning and take them off at night are quietly wondering what happened to that clear vision they once enjoyed. They are puzzled as to why they must continue to use glasses in order to see — and they are also inwardly concerned that these "corrective" devices get stronger and stronger as their eyes grow weaker and weaker over time.

Certainly, glasses can be a part of the solution when used carefully and consciously, but the real answer is to find the way to return to healthy, clear seeing as much as possible **with our own eyes.**

There is another, longer-sighted stance to take on the subject of vision! It's a view that liberates us from our old ways of thinking, seeing, and being ...

Joy Thompson

This is not the last word on vision by any stretch. This book offers a new hope and a new paradigm that is so much more exciting to invest in compared to the old one; the possibility of clearer vision and healthier eyes. Not just for the "lucky ones", but through education, for everyone.

Of course, no one should accept this at face value. Please read on and after reading, you might also begin to do some research of your own. My experience has been that in finding the answer to one of my questions, another question always comes to mind, and off I go again, searching for more answers!

Welcome to your first step towards moving to the other side of the fuzziness, into a world of improved clarity, inside and outside.

You have a right to see that well.

CHAPTER ONE

The Question That Changed My Life

"The most courageous act is still to think for yourself. Aloud."
— Coco Chanel

My Personal Story of Vision Lost and Regained

Almost all of my life I have experienced good vision. That is, I have been able to see clearly at all distances, without requiring glasses. I was an extremely active child — always outdoors playing games and sports. Although I had good reading skills, I was a light reader; reading perhaps one book per month, or even less. My young life was lived outside our house in the yard, fishing at our nearby creek, playing in the woods by the hour, constructing tree swings and forts, at the school-yard playing sports — that sort of thing.

I now realize that I was naturally far-sighted, but lucky enough to be able to focus at the near point — just not for long! Off I would go, losing interest in my books — outdoor adventures were calling me. I loved the sights in my outdoor world. I remember drinking in the fall colours in my home town and feeling the wonder in such a rich palette, climbing trees because the view from the higher branches was so delightful, and playing ball for countless hours, just for the fun and excitement of a good throw or a perfect catch.

In order to achieve in school I developed a very good memory for what was taught in class so I wouldn't have to review much in preparation for tests. Studying was such a drudge that kept me cloistered in my room, indoors, where I did not want to be! I couldn't study outside like a few of my friends, because in short order the books would be abandoned for play.

Right after I entered high school, when I was about 13 years old, I came home from school and complained to my Mother that my eyes "felt funny" a lot of the time. It almost hurt to keep my eyes on the books at school, but when I would look out the window the feeling would go away.

Mom thought I must need glasses and made an appointment with an Optometrist to get them. He placed me behind his big black contraption with all the lenses and asked me a lot of questions.

When he was finished, he called my Mom into the room and said, "This girl has an eye **muscle** problem. She doesn't need glasses, and don't let anybody put them on her! Her eye muscles need strengthening for seeing up close and I'm giving her a set of exercises and a prism to use for one month."

I owe so much to this man, but unfortunately I don't even remember his name. I have a very inquisitive nature and I was fascinated by the exercises he gave me. I did them faithfully every day for the month, by which time I could read and do schoolwork without the "funny feeling" coming back.

Obviously, my far-sightedness had increased by age 13 and the muscles that helped my eyes focus up close had weakened. The exercises the Optometrist gave me strengthened those muscles and that was all that was required for me to be seeing clearly up close, and being able to hold that focus, again.

Fast forward about 20 years and I was a young mother with a baby girl. I was very busy just learning the ropes of motherhood and getting settled into a new home. To add to the busy-ness of that time, I unwisely decided to take two very demanding university courses. So I was extremely busy all day and then, whenever the baby was sleeping, I was studying.

Like so many others, I took my eyesight for granted and I figured that as long as I could keep my eyes open they would work for me.

Late one night after the baby was sleeping and I had finished some sewing, I noticed that my right eye felt funny and seemed to have some kind of grey film over it. I rubbed it and splashed water on my face as I prepared to hit the books for a couple of hours. The eye was a little sore also, but I ignored that symptom too, and studied long into the night.

Next morning when I woke up, after a few minutes of sleepy disbelief, I realized that my right eye was completely blind. Looking out of my left eye only, everything was clear and normal. Looking only with my right eye, there was nothing but black-ness. With both eyes open I saw multiple and messy images of everything, since of course my brain had had no time at all to adjust to the situation.

To say I was terrified is such an understatement, but I'll leave out the rest of the drama, as there was a lot of it ...

On with the story. I was examined by a baffled Optometrist that day and then booked in to see a Neurologist two weeks later.

A very long and frightening two weeks it was, with no improvement at all in that eye. Finally I got a diagnosis of "optic neuritis", which is often a symptom of multiple sclerosis, but the doctor felt that "at least for now", I wasn't presenting MS. He said that the neuritis should clear up in about six months' time and I would have to cope as best I could until then.

And so I did ... but I still recall the terror and the incredible difficulty I experienced, just trying to live my life very minimally, during those months. My case of lost sight arrived just before Thanksgiving one year, and right on cue the next spring, my eye-sight fully returned over about a six week period.

I will also never, ever forget the joy of that spring! Every flower, every colour, every nuance of light and shadow that was again clear to me was cause for unbelievable celebration. And the icing on that cake was, of course, the sight of my daughter's beautiful face, without distortion, halos, multiple images or any remaining blur.

Hallelujah!

The benefit to me now is that I can empathize completely with anyone suffering from dramatically lowered vision, eye disease, visual distortion, double images — any of it — because one terrifying year, I experienced it all. I was beyond eye exercises, beyond natural vision improvement, beyond help, except for the help of having a condition that did heal over time, thank heaven. I was lucky.

That saying, "You don't know what you've got until you lose it" certainly applied to me, and it was a lesson well and thoroughly learned.

Optic neuritis is an inflammation of the optic nerve that may cause a complete (as in my case) or partial loss of vision in the affected eye.

The optic nerve carries messages from the retina of the eye and relays them to the visual cortex of the brain to be processed into visual images. Inflammation of the optic nerve causes loss of vision because of the swelling and destruction of the myelin sheath covering the optic nerve.

I vowed never to push myself so hard again. I dropped the university studies and spent my time enjoying the baby and my new home, making sure I got lots of rest! Really taking care of my health, which I had previously taken for granted, became and remained a high priority for me.

Moving forward in time about 12 more years … I had resumed my career as a teacher and 1995 was the year that I made a change from teaching Physical Education to regular classroom work.

It was also the year that I noticed that my reading vision was getting blurry. I hadn't been to an Optometrist in many years, since my vision had remained very good, but I made an appointment to see what was going on with my eyes.

In less than 15 minutes I had been examined and handed a prescription for reading glasses. Perhaps I shouldn't have been surprised, but I was.

I said something like:

"I've been marking a lot of papers and doing reports. I think my eyes are just tired and strained. Isn't there something I can do for this?"

The answer was short and sweet:

"Get these glasses and wear them."

I decided right away to get a second opinion and my next visit was with an Ophthalmologist. She gave me a slightly different prescription, but otherwise the conversation was the same as with the Optometrist, except that she added this prediction:

"Right now you just require reading glasses, but in a few years, you'll need bi-focals and then you can just wear glasses all the time. It's handier."

I said, "How do you know I will need bi-focals?"

Her not-so-comforting reply was, "That's just what commonly happens at your age. You are over forty now."

Not knowing what else to do, I got the prescription filled and wore the glasses for one week, by which time I realized that my eyes were already worse. Print that had been clear previously was fuzzy now that I was using the glasses. I spent a lot of time looking for them and soon understood why people might want glasses they could wear all the time. It saved looking for them!

However, a part of me kept repeating that something wasn't quite right. I began to understand that the glasses were not "corrective" lenses at all because they weren't correcting anything. I originally needed them in order to read small type — about 8 or 10 point type had become blurry for me — but after a couple of weeks of using glasses,

Joy Thompson

I needed them for 12 point type and sometimes even for 14 point, especially in dim lighting.

My vision was deteriorating even faster now that I was using the reading glasses; there was no question about it. When I talked to people I knew who wore glasses, many of them wearing bi-focals or tri-focals, they simply responded with something like, "Yeah, that's what happens. You get glasses and they get stronger and stronger and you need them more and more. Then in middle-age you get bi-focals or tri-focals because you need two or three different prescriptions for different distances. It's part of the aging process."

The answers I got about people's vision were always accompanied by a sense of defeat and a giving-in to what was inevitable. It was depressing, to say the least.

It was very clear to me that my glasses were just creating another problem, so I stopped wearing them and worked in only short stints with bright light, determined to find out what was really going on.

I kept thinking:

"If the rest of my body can heal when it is weakened or injured, why not my eyes?"

Meanwhile, there was another pair of eyes in my house that wasn't faring well at all. My baby girl, now grown to age 12, had been having trouble seeing in the distance; just the opposite problem to mine. She complained that the words on the blackboard were fuzzy, and on the soccer field or in the schoolyard it was hard for her to recognize shapes in the distance.

Off we went to another Optometrist. (I kept thinking that if I talked to different professionals, I might come across someone with a different viewpoint or someone who was at least willing to have a discussion with me about my concerns. I'm sorry to say that didn't happen.)

While in the Optometrist's waiting room with my daughter I stepped out to use the washroom. During the time that I was absent, she was taken into the examination room, her vision was measured, and she was standing back in the waiting room with a prescription for glasses in her hand.

I insisted on speaking with the Optometrist, but he gave me a very curt answer. "I've measured your daughter's vision. She needs glasses. Get the prescription filled and get her to wear them. So, that will be all for today ..." and I was ushered out.

I knew that my daughter had been under some stress at school and was spending longer and longer times reading in her room or playing on our new family computer and I *just knew* this was the cause of her vision problems. I had trouble accepting that a child who could see perfectly clearly a few months before would now have to wear glasses all the time.

Forever? At age 12, was this vision "correction" a "life sentence" for my child?

Something wasn't right. I knew that there was something about this whole "eye thing" that I needed to understand, and I was determined to find out what it was, with or without the help of the "experts".

Meanwhile, my daughter needed glasses in order to see at school. Over the next two years her prescription was increased twice, landing at -3.50 and -3.25, and she wore glasses all the time, except for reading.

I was struggling away, using my reading glasses only as a last resort, doing close work for short periods, determined to rest my strained eyes as much as possible. I certainly didn't want to repeat my "optic neuritis" experience or something even worse.

These were "pre-Google" days and I found no help in my public library, but the many questions I was asking kept percolating in my mind ...

Help on the Horizon

As luck would have it, being a teacher, I belonged to the Ontario Institute for Studies in Education, and a brochure appeared in the mail the winter of 1995/96, describing an upcoming seminar on "Natural Vision Improvement" that would be led by Elizabeth Abraham, a Natural Vision Improvement Teacher, and held in Toronto.

"Learn methods of improving eyesight" it claimed. I was ecstatic! Even though it was a two-hour drive from my home and I drove through a horrible winter storm to get there, I was determined to learn what this woman was teaching.

The seminar was fascinating and very informative. The information I heard that night opened the doors for me and things clicked into place. I knew I was on the way to finding the answers I craved.

From Elizabeth Abraham, I learned that evening about Dr. William Bates and the pioneering work that led to the field of NVI (Natural Vision Improvement). She talked about the causes of near- and far-sightedness and the "Bates Method" that was developed to restore eyes to healthy seeing again. She outlined the issue of dependency on lenses, and how so often it is this very dependency that creates a downward spiral into worse and worse vision, over time.

I knew this to be true from both my experience and the deterioration of eyesight I was witnessing in my daughter. Finally, I was getting some answers!

That evening, Elizabeth taught us methods of relaxation, so critical for healthy eyes, and then basic exercises intended to stimulate our visual systems and get our eyes working dynamically again.

I went home and for three weeks I religiously followed the practices and exercises for far-sightedness outlined in the seminar, every single day, and I was rewarded with clear vision restored! This was reminiscent for me of that time all those years ago when the Optometrist in my home town was so extremely helpful. I simply did the exercises and my eyes responded.

I could not contain my glee, and everyone near me heard about all I was learning and experiencing. I wanted to share my good news with everyone and to inspire them to liberate themselves from glasses and that depressing mind-set regarding the inevitability of eyes deteriorating over time. I knew for sure that there was another and much more optimistic way to look at this whole situation.

And what could be more important than seeing well and taking care of our eyes? A quick flashback to my optic neuritis episode kept reminding me that assuredly, this was a subject of high importance for everyone.

It was exhilarating! The glasses I had so obediently purchased had only that one-week term on my nose, and I was back to seeing clearly again (and I still see that well, eighteen years later).

It is part of my nature to ask questions and I had many more:

"What causes loss of vision?"

"Is there more to how we see than just the physical factors?"

"Why do so many people think it's normal to need to wear glasses in order to see?"

"Wouldn't healthy eyes, by definition, see well?"

"Do healthy eyes develop eye diseases or could eye disease be the result of eyes being unhealthy (not seeing well) for many years?"

"What about bi- or tri-focal lenses? Wouldn't they be hard on the brain and body, looking through them and the two or three different corrections there?"

"Hasn't anybody else asked these questions?"

The answers I found to these and more questions in those early weeks and months just fueled my desire to understand more. I was obsessed, and read everything I could find on the subject.

Dr. William Bates and the studies he did in New York in the 1920's and the conclusions he found are as relevant and important to our understanding of eyes and vision now as they were back then. And yet, he and his findings were dismissed by the medical establishment with a metaphorical wave of the hand.

It took little research on my part, however, to discover that the basic "Bates Method" works … and to realize that these practices remain the real and practical solution for blurry eyesight and unhealthy eyes.

Vision Educators today have adapted and developed the basic Bates Method to use with those who have a long-standing dependency on lenses, for people with very healthy eyes, and for everyone in between. It does take some time and patience to return to clearer seeing, but the rewards are amazing and so heartening!

When these practices are taught early, to young people, the need for that first pair of glasses can often be eliminated while eyesight is strengthened and kept strong through simple methods.

After I had improved my own vision and learned a great deal about William Bates and his teachings, I convinced my then 13-year-old daughter, Gwen, that the prescription lenses she was wearing were not helping the situation at all. By that time she was wearing contacts a lot of the time as well as glasses.

She didn't want to wear glasses to school, so I created a program for her that worked with the situation as it was. By this time, I knew I wanted to teach Vision Education to others and I needed some of my own experience to help me learn just how it was done.

The compromise I worked out with Gwen was that she could wear her contact lenses to school and then remove them when she arrived home, spending the evening without lenses at all as much as possible. She had a moderate prescription, so going without lenses and looking at her blurry world was certainly a challenge in the beginning.

Gwen was cooperative, however, about doing the exercises and particularly the relaxation practices I suggested, which she loved. She could feel the tension in her eyes dissipating with these simple exercises.

Soon, as her distance vision slowly began to improve, she felt a discomfort that she articulated … "Sometimes it feels kind of scary to see so far away and I feel like I want to look down or read a book or do something, to stop looking and seeing."

We talked about these feelings and slowly her confidence grew. She also commented one day to me that she felt like her glasses had "protected" her, and she felt "wide open" without them. Noticing this seemed to help her resolve the issue as she moved into clearer and clearer vision.

Six months later Gwen's prescription was reduced to less than half what it was when we began, and she was very comfortable in most situations, without lenses.

I will never forget one Saturday morning when she was lying on my bed and we were talking. She looked over at my dresser where there were several bottles of perfume, and she said, "You know, six months ago when I looked at your dresser without my glasses, all I saw was a big blur. Now I can see the perfume bottles and I can even read the labels on them!"

It was so gratifying to see her accomplishment in the form of new (lighter) prescriptions! Now we had a record of the changes in her vision. We had Optometrists' prescriptions that documented her progress to stronger lenses and we also had prescriptions that showed her improvement all the way back to clarity.

Gwen was proud of her accomplishment and she put together a very impressive "How I Improved My Vision" display for the Science Fair and won third prize in the county.

I am a natural born teacher, and I was just so eager to teach all that I had learned to other teachers, imagining the benefits to children in our classrooms, learning how to preserve and care for their eyes and eyesight. I happily put on a presentation at the next Teacher's Professional Day.

I summed up by saying, "We teach young children how to care for their skin, teeth, hair, and how to maintain healthy bodies and eat nutritiously, but we don't teach them anything at all about how to care for their eyes and prevent problems. What could be more important? And it's all so easy!" I declared, and everyone seemed to agree.

I also taught yoga at various locations in the area, and I told my yoga students about what I was learning and taught several of the simple vision practices as part of my classes. Everyone was appreciative, but some of my students, who suffered from chronic eye problems and seriously impaired vision, asked me to take them on as "projects". This was a delight to me, and I worked with anyone interested, creating a plan and program for them to improve their eyesight. I didn't ask for any fee at the time, because I wanted to have these experiences as part of my learning.

The results were exciting! Students were reducing their dependency on lenses and learning to relax even more deeply than through yoga alone. William Bates taught that if our eyes are not relaxed our bodies cannot fully relax either, so in improving their ability to rest their visual systems my students were beginning to experience much deeper states of relaxation overall. Many people reported to me that not only were their eyes feeling and functioning better, but they were feeling better all over!

Comments and results like these encouraged me to no end and I was hooked. I knew I wanted passionately to become a Vision Educator and teach this to anyone interested.

I made an appointment with Elizabeth Abraham in Toronto, and asked her how I could receive training in Vision Education. Following her advice to get as much experience with different schools of thought as possible, I studied in several different locations over the next two years. My quest took me to western Canada, California and Spain. I read every book I could find on the subject and continued working with anyone interested, for nothing, and then later for a very nominal fee.

Every single time that someone committed to the relaxation practices and exercises on a regular basis, we saw results. People were able to reduce their dependency on lenses, or eliminate the need for lenses altogether, and most importantly, stop the downward spiral of needing stronger and stronger prescription glasses or contacts.

(To be thorough, I have to mention that some people who showed interest actually wouldn't take the time, or thought they didn't have the time, for the natural practices I gave them, and of course the process didn't work for them.)

This whole process can be compared to someone starting an exercise program at a gym to improve cardiovascular health and body strength. If the person shows up on a regular basis and follows the program, they will see results, of course. No one can say how fast or how far they can take it, but changes will occur.

It's exactly the same for a healthy vision regimen. If we are are willing to do it, we will be rewarded with clearer vision and healthier eyes and we will feel it subjectively as well as having measurable results.

If a child sprains his leg, we don't say, "Oh, that's too bad. Your legs are weaker now but you can use crutches to get around for the rest of your life."

Does that sound ridiculous? It's not much more ridiculous than the throngs of people walking around in our society who went through a bad patch, got glasses, and are wearing them for life!

Nowadays, we have a surgical "quick fix" on offer as well. People are having their eyes "lasered" at ever-increasing rates. Laser surgery clinics are highly competitive businesses that must make a bottom line in order to survive. Whether we have our eyes "done" at a high price, or get them altered "on special" at some reduced rate, there are real risks to laser surgery, and there is no "quick fix" available if something goes wrong.

Of course, laser surgery, just like lenses, does nothing to correct the root of the problem which is tension and lack of dynamics in a weakened visual system. Once this is restored, the eye (an incredibly sophisticated, adaptable mechanism) will begin to heal and correct itself.

Most of us agree that eyesight is a precious commodity. I believe that if everyone understood the basic principles of eye health and the natural alternative to stronger lenses and surgery, they would try the risk-free option first.

And that is the whole reason for this book; to get the alternative out there, front and centre, so that people can make informed and powerful decisions that serve them and their desire for health.

When we strive for health, our eyes and vision must be included!

CHAPTER TWO

Sweet Inspiration

"Few men are willing to brave the disapproval of their fellows, the censure of their colleagues, the wrath of their society. Moral courage is a rarer commodity than bravery in battle or great intelligence. Yet it is the one essential, vital quality for those who seek to change a world that yields most painfully to change."
— Bobby Kennedy

Dr. William Horatio Bates (1860 - 1931)

Thank goodness that Dr. William Bates had the courage to believe that a healthier approach was worth investigating and pursuing. He bravely asked the questions listed in Chapter One, and many more.

He realized that, working as an Eye Physician and Surgeon in New York City in the 1920's, he was rarely seeing improved results. He observed his patients' eyesight getting weaker and weaker; lenses prescribed which were stronger and stronger as time went by, and he was alarmed at the increase in eye disease.

Bates wanted to help people get healthier, not just observe them becoming more and more ill. In his pursuit of some solid answers to the problem of weakening eyes and vision, he closed a lucrative Ophthalmology practice in pursuit of the answers.

Over four years, Bates examined many thousands of eyes under a myriad of different circumstances, carefully recording all his observations. Bates meticulously researched and discovered the underlying causes for weakened eyesight and eyes.

He used all his new data to develop specific approaches to bring eyes back to a much healthier state; "The Bates Method" as it has come to be known.

We have six extra-ocular muscles holding our eyes in place and these muscles are responsible for eye movement in their voluntary capacity. They are the muscles we use consciously when moving our eyes.

However, Bates discovered that the tiny muscles supporting our eyes have another, involuntary job to do as well. They also are able to actually change the shape of the eyeball, making it elongate so that we can see things up close, or relax, so that the eyeball will assume a "flatter" shape, enabling us to see in the distance.

And so, when someone stares at the computer screen for hours on end or reads continually, those muscles encircling the eye must constantly be flexed. Eventually, they may become "stuck" in flex mode and when we look away from our books or computers, we discover that in the distance, things look fuzzy.

(Working on this book, if I get carried away writing and ignore my own advice for a couple of hours, I prove to myself that this is true, because when I finally step away from my work, I find that I am near-sighted! Thank heaven I know how to correct that, and I also know better than to allow myself to become so absorbed by my work without taking any breaks, too often.)

Bates discovered in his observations that when the mind tenses (as in struggling to understand or because of emotional stressors), the eye muscles tighten. This tightening is of course what pulls the eyes off focus and causes vision to blur. So impaired vision is generally the result of two types of tension combined; mental and physical.

Less than one-quarter of students beginning a computer course at the college level are near-sighted, but by graduation over three-quarters of them are, and are wearing corrective lenses. This is the simple result of studying and doing close work for three years without any practices to counter-act the affect of all that on the eyes. (Doesn't that sound like some "proof" of Bates' theory?)

Bates worked towards creating a state of what he called "dynamic relaxation" where the eye is active and involved while it does the work of seeing in a very relaxed way. This is the way babies and young children see naturally and is the ideal state that we in Vision Education strive for.

At the opposite end of the scale, we have those who are having trouble seeing up close. Their eye muscles have weakened and cannot flex and hold, so reading printed material or computer screens isn't easy at all. This is when we are typi-cally told, as I was, that we need our "first pair" of reading glasses.

Bates contended that what is happening here is that the muscles are unfit and weakened, so they cannot contract. That doesn't need to be the end of the story, however. There are ways to strengthen these extra-ocular muscles and get our eyes to focus easily at the close point. That's what I did at age 13, and did again after turning 40, with great success.

Some argue that the lens is involved in focusing, and that the lens hardens as we age. To address this question, Bates actually removed the lens from a patient's eye and observed the eye, reshaping itself and focusing with no lens in place at all. Certainly, the lens plays a necessary part of our focusing mechanism and our ability to see detail, but we can also affect its functioning with specific, targeted practices.

When we relax our eyes fully, our entire nervous system relaxes. This is a mental, physical and emotional phenomenon. Having practiced eye relaxation for many years, I can attest that this is true as can many of my clients … as we feel our eyes relaxing (and this is a learned skill), we learn to become aware as our entire body follows suit.

And so, to keep our bodies and eyes functioning at their best and in a relaxed way, we have to understand that our eyes do not function independently of our bodies and brain; that all components are part and parcel of the whole system.

Bates observed consistently that once we are using glasses regularly, the healthy dynamics of the eyes stop, because the glasses are doing the refractive work for us. Our eyes weaken while the glasses do the work of focusing for us.

Those people who have been ready to hear and implement the message of Natural Vision Improvement methods have a strong knowing that their eyesight can be strengthened and they have been ready to take that step.

My eighteen years of passionate experience with this subject has brought me to the strong belief that we need to get "care of the eyes" moved forward in our consciousness and viewed in a new and powerful way. In a very short time, anyone can understand how to care for their eyes and their functioning in general, how to prevent computer eyestrain and other visual stresses, and how to rest their eyes deeply and stimulate them in ways that help to keep them healthy.

It may appear to be normal to wear glasses or contacts since over 50% of our adult population does this, but it is not natural or healthy to wear prescription glasses all the time. All we have to do is "step outside of the box" long enough to see the simplicity and sensibility of the natural approach.

If we can imagine that William Bates was correct in his assertion that stress and tension are factors that contribute to impaired vision, then it logically follows that lenses and surgery are not necessarily "correcting" anything, but rather are providing a way for us to manage with eyes that are unwell.

And we are not managing too well, judging by the number of people buying stronger and stronger lenses, opting for laser surgery, often more than once, and developing eye diseases at younger and younger ages.

What if, seeing more clearly *with our own eyes, naturally,* was healthier at every level? Would it be worth it to us to experience healthy eyes that use the light efficiently, and allow the full spectrum of light frequency to pass into our bodies? (Keep in mind that eyes are the only part of our bodies designed to let light in.)

For spiritual seekers like me, light is more than just the stuff you need in order to find something. Light is synonymous with goodness and knowledge and wisdom, and we see the spiritual masters and great leaders as those who brought light into the world and imparted knowledge to guide us to see in all ways.

To some of us, eyes are sacred territory. Anyone who has really, truly connected with another living being through eye contact knows this, and knows that they are not to be covered over with glass for decades or submitted to laser cuts and techniques. They are to be studied, understood, encouraged, respected and treated with care and gentleness, for life.

As Bates proved that it was the combination of physical and mental tension and overall weakness that resulted in blurry vision and unhealthy eyes, our task lies in undoing this chronic state of tension. We need to teach our eyes the delicate art of relaxation, and we do that partly by working with the involuntary muscles. That was Bates' brilliance; his method of getting to the heart of what we habitually were doing involuntarily and making it conscious, through re-training.

The paradox is that once we've re-trained our eyes to work the way they were designed to work, the healthy habits we've adopted go back to being involuntary, and everything works in sync once again.

Health at all levels is indeed our natural state. Our health is not the responsibility of the doctors or surgeons. It's our individual responsibility to take health into our own hands; to study the facts, understand what our eyes and bodies require, and then to follow through.

Based on my own experience and so many others I've observed, I'm willing to guarantee that the results are a million times worth the small effort required.

It is a sad and sorry thing that Bates was not taken more seriously by his peers. Not agreeing with all he presented would be fine; even disagreeing with his methodology and calling it "unscientific" in its method probably has some validity as well. However, ignoring the fact that so many people have been getting results with the "Bates method" or using some part of it to gain improved visual health, just doesn't make any sense at all.

There is something to be learned from all the work that Bates did, and all that has followed in the wake of what he discovered about eyes. Dr. Bates' book, "Better Eyesight Without Glasses" is still available and has stood the test of time.

Let's have a look at a few people who began with the Bates method and experienced dramatic results. I'm giving a brief outline here of the stories of each of these contributors, but their works are still available for anyone interested to pursue.

Meir Schneider

I have often described Meir Schneider to people as a "walking, seeing miracle" because his story is certainly one that blows any accepted beliefs about what is possible, sky high.

Meir was born blind.

By the age of seven, after a few surgical attempts to repair his eyes, he was declared legally blind and incurable by his doctors.

Meir had trouble accepting this "life sentence" and at the age of seventeen, he began to work with the Bates Method and a variety of other natural techniques and slowly his vision began to emerge. Within four years, he was able to read, to see and to function, and he was, and still is, far from blind!

Early on, I was deeply touched, reading Meir's autobiography, "Self-Healing: My Life and Vision". It truly is a story of heroic individualism, determination, and enlightenment on a number of levels.

It's important to remember that if one human being can achieve those kinds of results, lots of possibilities are open to the rest of us, and no situation necessarily deserves the label of "hopeless" or the depressing statement, "That's just the way it is; what can you do?"

My answer to that kind of attitude is, "Something can always help or give hope and possibly bring results. Why not do something that just might open the door for improvement to arrive?"

What do we have to gain by arguing for limitations rather than possibilities?

Meir Schneider has developed his own method of self-healing and he teaches people to be pro-active in their own health with a regimen of exercise, movement, deep breathing, mental imagery, self-massage, and other techniques.

Meir is a very dramatic example, but the world is full of examples of people who have taken a different approach from the mainstream answer and have improved their eyesight through safe and natural methods. I have done so, my daughter, and the hundreds of people I have worked with over the years. Add to this all the success stories to be heard from Natural Vision Educators all over the globe, and there is a strong case for the validity of this approach.

What is required is a belief in the body's ability to heal itself, and a listening to that voice inside each one of us that believes in possibilities. We also, I will re-state, need to take our healing into our own hands; following others' (including doctors') advice when it feels just right to us, and throwing it out the window when it doesn't.

Barring any physical accidents having occurred, we each have all the equipment we require for clear seeing. We just need to learn how to work with it. Because the healing is natural and therefore takes some time, observation and patience and the ability to take some pleasure in the journey is required.

Margaret Corbett

Margaret Darst Corbett met Dr. William H. Bates after consulting him about her husband's eyesight. She was so interested in his approach that she became his pupil, and eventually taught his methods of Vision Education in her Los Angeles "School of Eye Education" in the 1930's and 40's.

Mrs. Corbett is the author of "Help Yourself to Better Sight", a very practical book that I refer to frequently.

Corbett was highly criticized by the establishment and finally taken to court for "practicing medicine without a license" but was subsequently acquitted. She demonstrated that she was working as an educator, teaching the basic Bates method to those who were interested in learning.

Many of her students came forward in the court-room at the time to tell their stories of improved vision, using the practices being taught to them by Mrs. Corbett.

One of Corbett's more famous students was the science fiction writer, Aldous Huxley.

Aldous Huxley

Aldous Huxley, the well-known author of the science fiction novel, *Brave New World* and many others, had very low vision when he began to study the Bates method with Margaret Corbett in the 1930's.

Huxley's eyesight improved and he wrote an enlightening book on the subject called "The Art of Seeing" which chronicles his experience and outlines a route to follow for those who believe in natural health and consider eyeglasses unnatural.

I think it's interesting that a science fiction writer would become one of our visionaries when it comes to visual health. It came naturally to Huxley to open his mind to new possibilities and ideas. Having the opportunity to affect his healing himself obviously appealed to him and worked for him. I imagine it was easy for him to think "outside the box" since that's where his story ideas came from anyway.

Through working with Margaret Corbett, Huxley became aware of his many unhealthy (and unconscious) habits of seeing. For one simple example, he discovered that he had a habit of staring unblinkingly. He learned to move his eyes in a healthy way, to blink lots and through this, keep his eyes lubricated and stimulated. Once he practiced moving and blinking his eyes on a regular basis, he created healthy unconscious habits once again. "The Art of Seeing" is testimony to Huxley's restored visual health; first published in 1942 and still available.

Bates' work was complete in the 1930's and results comparable to Huxley's were reported often, and have continued to be, from that time on. William Bates created the spark that has inspired so many of us to keep working with his "method" or derivations of it.

Although mainstream thought is that because his studies didn't meet the criteria required to make them acceptable as "science" many people are seeing better and better using these practices ... and certainly, this is inspirational, good news!

Something for all of us to celebrate and learn from.

CHAPTER THREE

The Basics

**"It's not what you look at that matters.
It's what you see."**
— *Henry David Thoreau*

Many wise leaders and writers have long extolled the beauty and the key importance of our eyes; the "windows of the soul" as Shakespeare proclaimed. All of the great spiritual masters, when depicted in art, are shown with beautiful, light-filled and mesmerizing eyes.

These charismatic leaders are seeing with their hearts, their whole bodies and brain, and their intuition all at the same time. They are able to see the big picture as well as the details, the focal point and the periphery, and that is why when they speak, their talk absorbs and arrests us.

Their very healthy and glowing eyes are made of the same material as all the other eyes in the world. We all have the same equipment — in most cases, perfectly functioning equipment — when we are born.

With some effort and understanding we can bring these structures to the best functioning possible. By paying attention to how we feel when we look, we learn more and more about our full connection to seeing.

All the Equipment You Need

Before we go further, let's just take a minute to identify some of the "key players" in seeing and look at how they function before we get into some basic exercises and practices. We'll move from front to back in our eyes' structure.

Cornea:

The cornea is the front surface of the eye which is there to protect all the inner structures. The cornea affects the angle at which the light enters the eye and it is nourished, conditioned and soothed by blinking and by tears. The tear ducts are tucked up above the centre of the eye and every time we blink, we supply this amazingly healthy and protective fluid to our cornea to help it in its protective function.

Pupil:

That black hole in the centre of your iris is your pupil. This is where light enters the body. The pupil appears to expand and contract according to light intensity, appearing larger in darkness and smaller in response to light, but it is actually the activity of the iris that changes the appearance of the pupil. A pupil that appears enlarged can also signal emotional excitement.

Iris:

The iris is the coloured part of the eye and is named for Iris, the Greek goddess of the rainbow. The iris is actually a diaphragm that changes size in response to light. This beautiful feature embodies very distinctive, highly individualized colours and patterns; streaks, lines, dots, and swirls, which make each eye beautiful and completely distinct from all others.

Lens:

Behind the pupil is the lens. Along with the cornea, it helps to refract light to be focused on the retina.

Movement and response of the lens is important to clear vision.

Ciliary Muscle:

The ciliary muscle is a layer of smooth muscle that controls our ability to view objects at varying distances. It has an affect on the shape of the lens.

Sclera:

The white part of the eye. The sclera supports and holds other structures in place. Stressed sclera will be "bloodshot"; this is an early warning sign of visual stress.

Extra-ocular Muscles:

Six muscles hold the eye in its orbit and are attached to the sclera. The recti muscles are above, below, at the left and right side of each eye, and the oblique muscles are in the corners. Without stimulation, these muscles become unfit and rigid but do respond to exercise, massage and relaxation. With some experience, it's easy to begin to discern subjectively when eyes are relaxed and refreshed, as compared to stressed and fatigued.

Aqueous Humour:

This is a clear fluid that fills the space between the cornea and the front of the vitreous humour. It maintains intra-ocular pressure and inflates the globe of the eye.

Vitreous Humour:

The vitreous is a jelly-like substance between the retina and the lens, which creates the shape of the eyeball.

Retina:

The curved back of the eyeball; an extremely delicate area made of rod and cone cells which receive the light and communicate images to the brain through the optic nerve.

Macula:

The macula is the oval-shaped, highly pigmented yellow spot near the centre of the retina. It absorbs excess blue and ultraviolet light that enters the eye and acts as a natural sunblock.

Fovea:

The fovea is a small depression in the centre of the macula where clear vision occurs. The fovea has the largest concentration of cone cells and is responsible for high resolution, central vision.

Rods:

Photoreceptor cells, responsible for detail seeing: they are extremely light sensitive.

Cones:

Cones are colour receptors, requiring more light in order to function. More cones are found in the macula of the retina.

Optic Nerve:

The optic nerve brings the blood and nerve supply from the brain to the eye. It receives images from the eye and transports them to the brain for interpretation.

Choroid:

The choroid is the part of the eye that supplies nourishment for the retina.

The Basics of Natural Vision Improvement

Here are the basic elements of a Natural Vision Improvement program.

1. Rest and Relaxation

Eyes are meant to see in a relaxed fashion. We must learn to relax our eyes and to recognize how that feels. This awareness helps us to notice any tension in our seeing mechanism.

2. Remove Lenses

In order for us to become aware of what we are really seeing, we need to remove lenses in safe situations, on a regular basis. Wearing a reduced prescription can also help with the transition to clearer seeing. We need to reduce our dependency on the stronger lenses and that means being "in the blur" at least some of the time.

Pinhole glasses can sometimes be very helpful as part of any vision improvement program. They are non-prescription lenses that are made of hard plastic, including the "lens" area, which is dotted with tiny, evenly spaced holes all across the front. These holes help to introduce light to the eye in an organized fashion, thus making it easier for the eye to focus. They can be used regularly in safe situations, to stimulate the eyes to see while making the process easier.

3. Stimulating the Eyes with Full-Spectrum Light

Our eyes are often subjected to electric lighting, which is usually missing the full daylight spectrum, although better quality full-spectrum lighting is available if we look for it.

In NVI, we have practices that use the great quality of outdoor light to stimulate the eyes. Natural light stimulates the retina and soothes the optic nerve. This high quality light nourishes and calms our bodies as well.

4. Using Specific Exercises

This is when Vision Improvement becomes more personalized. Sometimes one eye is "weaker" than another and needs some specific stimulation. In this step, we "listen" to the eyes and their needs.

No pair of eyes on the planet is exactly the same as another, so we need to listen to them individually while encouraging them to work as a "team". We want to have both eyes working at the same power, or as close as possible. Since the left eye activates the right brain, and the right eye activates the left brain, we want to be "looking" with our whole brains! Otherwise, looking through one much clearer-seeing eye all day, every day, gets things off balance. It is much more authentic to have glasses off and working at close to the same power. Once both eyes are actively participating in seeing (rather than passively, as when the glasses are on), intuition gets sharper. This is something my clients notice often as their eyes strengthen and cooperate better ... it's a feeling of being more "tuned in" that accompanies the results, and is cause for celebration.

5. Evaluating Nutritional Needs and Supplementation

Our eye/brain combination requires roughly 25% of the total nutrient requirement for our bodies. For growing children it is critically important that they get a diet rich in nutrients with supplements for the basics if necessary. A full accounting of all the nutrients required by the eyes and their sources is in the section on Children's Vision.

6. Maintenance Care

Some practices are necessarily part of a healthy lifestyle and eye program. Everyone should be familiar with the practice of palming which can be employed daily to refresh the eyes and keep them rested and therefore seeing in a relaxed manner. Relaxing the eyes regularly with some sort of swaying practice helps to guard against eyes getting tense and remaining so. Getting outside for brisk exercise under full-spectrum light on a daily basis is essential for clear vision and overall health.

We simply cannot stare at iphones, ipads, video games, computers, etc. for hours on end and have healthy eyes! What we can easily do, however, is take regular breaks from these gadgets and go over to a window or outdoors and gaze off into the far distance, allowing our eyes to relax. Breathe deeply, and the body will follow suit.

Technology can be fascinating and mesmerizing, but we need to be the ones in charge of how we use it and manage our time in a healthy way ... more about all of this later.

Many people have a nightly habit of climbing into bed to read before falling asleep; actually, I've had clients often tell me that they cannot fall asleep otherwise.

At the end of each day, our eyes are tired, and sitting to read after dark simply makes them exhausted, which is a habit we need to drop. Try light exercise like yoga or tai chi, or listening to music, a bath, or some other relaxing activity that doesn't require your eyes working so hard. Reserve earlier times in the day for reading, under good light, with rested eyes.

CHAPTER FOUR

Breaking out of the Box

"People who say it cannot be done should not interrupt those who are doing it."
— *George Bernard Shaw*

The paradigm that exists all around us regarding vision is huge and a bit mysterious. Even the very highly health-conscious, or people who know that their lifestyle is damaging their vision, or doctors who are supposedly committed to wellness, often seem to have an invisible wall around them when speaking about eyesight and the concept of improving it.

I experienced this "invisible wall" right after I improved my own vision in '96. I made an appointment with another Optometrist and went in for an examination. We went through the full examination, but this time I passed with flying colours, as I expected.

He remarked, "Your vision is excellent. You don't need any correction."

I beamed at him and then proudly explained that I had needed glasses just a few months before, and I showed him the dated prescription. Then I talked about the Natural Vision Improvement seminar and William Bates and the exercises I had done so faithfully, bringing me back to good vision again.

He looked right at me for the first time and said, "Yes, I've heard of the Bates Method, but there is absolutely no evidence that it works."

I said, "I'm sitting right here and now you know that it does work! If it works for me, it could obviously work for other people." With that remark, our exchange was ended and I was shown to the outer office where I paid for the examination and left, completely baffled.

Weren't Optometrists interested in people having good vision?

Wasn't a woman who clearly had improved her eyesight within the space between those examinations at least some proof that these practices could have an effect?

Was it really so impossible to entertain another, and to my view, much healthier, way of looking at eyes and eyesight?

Christine

I have had a multitude of experiences over the years that have encouraged me to just keep moving forward with this, regardless of popular opinion. One of those occurrences was the first time I gave a talk at a health foods market in Vancouver.

The young woman who scheduled my talk was bubbling over with enthusiasm for healthy living and learning. She had heard about what I was doing through a very enthusiastic client, so called about scheduling me to be one of their speakers at their monthly free talks.

The night arrived and I was greeted by Christine, who was lovely, and her effervescence shone through her stylish glasses. She explained that they expected a crowd and she showed me to the room where I would speak, which was completely set up and ready.

As I began speaking, I encouraged everyone to remove their glasses. I explained that they would remain comfortably seated, but I wanted their eyes to relax into "what they really saw" with their own eyes for awhile, and that I would be teaching some relaxation practices that they would be doing with lenses removed. I quickly noticed that Christine, seated in the back row, removed her glasses, but wasn't looking at all happy about it.

Of course, I added that if the thought of listening without their glasses on was too uncomfortable for them, they could leave them on. About half the people took their glasses off, which is about what I have come to expect.

The presentation lasted about two hours and this was a group of people who were totally committed to doing whatever they could, by natural means, to improve and guard their health, so I was in my element. We did many of the basic practices together as I was describing how the process worked. I concluded the talk by saying that I would be happy to stay behind for more discussion, one-on-one.

As I was thanking everyone, I noticed with my peripheral vision that Christine had left her back row seat and walked up to stand beside me, ready to speak herself. As I turned to look at her, I noticed her beautiful eyes, still without lenses.

She beamed. (She was very good at that! She had the kind of smile that radiated joy to everyone around her). She thanked me for my talk, presented me with a gift, and then added:

"I want everyone here to know that I've been wearing glasses full-time since I got them in high school, eight years ago. I took my glasses off tonight at the beginning of Joy's talk, and as I watched and listened and participated from the back of the room, I've noticed that everything has been getting clearer and clearer through the evening. I realize I've been doing something habitually that I just don't need to do anymore. I'll keep my glasses handy in case I need them, but from now on I'm going to see with my own eyes, and practice what I've learned here."

That was it for Christine! She had a fairly mild prescription; the same correction in both eyes with no other complications. She was extremely healthy; eating and living well, and it seemed the time was just right to simply let her eyes catch up.

I talked with Christine again about one year later, when I came back to speak at the market. She told me that she had never worn her glasses since that night, and after six months she was tested and the stipulation for wearing glasses for driving had been removed from her license. She was doing the basic practices on a daily basis and she loved them.

We both smiled and beamed at each other, eye to eye. Improving vision is certainly not always this simple and straightforward, but sometimes it is, and it's wonderful to witness.

Daniel's Story

When I met him in May of 2012, Daniel had the demeanor of a defeated man. He said he had "never heard of this", referring to the field of Natural Vision Improvement, but he was willing to try anything that would give him hope of improving his very limited vision.

Daniel had been very near-sighted all his life, and at the young age of 28, his vision worsened and he was diagnosed with "something like" retinitis pigmentosa. The doctors simply weren't sure what was causing his deteriorating vision. He definitely exhibited many of the symptoms of retinitis pigmentosa; poor night vision, loss of peripheral vision, light sensitivity, reduced visual field, slow adjustment to different light environments, poor colour separation, and extreme fatigue.

Daniel lost his job working on a ferry boat due to this diagnosis and as he began to draw unemployment insurance benefits, he felt more and more depressed about his situation.

He applied for other jobs and was less than honest with his employers about his eyesight, knowing that he wouldn't secure any kind of labourer's work if the employers were aware of his vision problems. He did find work, and managed as best he could over the next decade, living in the frightening shadow of what appeared to be impending blindness. Daniel was examined and diagnosed by several doctors, but was never offered anything that he might be able to do to improve his situation or soothe his ailing eyes.

Together, Daniel and I agreed to gently challenge things and we began to stimulate and relax his eyes through Vision Improvement methods. The first time I measured Daniel's vision, he could read only the top (largest) line on my eye chart, standing very close, at a distance of three feet from the chart.

Daniel performed the relaxation practices I gave him about twice as much as I had recommended, loving the feeling of surrender that would flood through his eyes and body as he went deeper and deeper into that soothing state. I gave him specific self-massage practices that would help reduce the extreme tension around his eyes.

I then began adding specific exercises weekly, designed to stimulate his peripheral vision and improve his distance seeing.

Exactly one month later, Daniel was able to read down four lines on my eye chart, standing at a distance of three feet. Both of us were astonished at his amazing progress and the world that was literally opening back up in front of him!

As I mentioned, Daniel had appeared to be (understandably) depressed and defeated when we began our work together. That day one month later, after measuring his vision, was the first time I saw him smile — one of those fabulous moments I'll never forget.

Daniel and I worked together for one year, noting every single bit of progress he was making, and celebrating each step. His energy and confidence were returning and it was wonderful for me to be a part of this transformation.

Then one day Daniel talked about all the problems he was having distinguishing colours; blues, purples and greens especially seemed to look all the same to him.

Once again, we decided to challenge the idea that nothing could be done. I went off to my local paint store and came home with many colour samples; bits of every colour and hue and tint, and I made him a colour puzzle.

Daniel's job was to look at a paint sample and then find its description on a chart; matching "sky blue" or "crimson red" with the corresponding sample. In the beginning, he was getting two or three colours correct out of 20, but after about four months he was scoring 18 out of 20 or higher on his "colour game".

We have continued to work with this, exploring all the different hues and tints I can find at the paint store (surprisingly, no one has yet asked me about my obsession with paint chips!) The more we worked with colour, the more Daniel learned to distinguish it. Now I would wager that he knows the names of colours better than most men. Some days he'll mention colours he's seen ... "I saw a house that was periwinkle blue yesterday", or, "I bought a lemon yellow shirt!" He's delighted to tell me these things and I love hearing them!

All we did here was challenge an accepted paradigm and the results have been, and continue to be, delightful. Just because Daniel had lost his ability to distinguish colour didn't, apparently, mean that that ability was forever lost. We just kept tweaking and tweaking, and he relearned how to see and distinguish colour, just as he had relearned so many other visual skills. He is continuing to this day, to improve and awaken his eyes.

And — and I believe this is a critical point — because his despair has lifted, he has become interested in a subjective way in what's going on. He is a keen and careful observer of how he sees.

This was a complete new lease on life for Daniel, who is still quite young at age 39. He subsequently decided to take a training course that requires lots of reading and writing and study, and he's the happiest student I know!

"Bring it on!" he says. "I can see it all!"

A couple of other little post-scripts about Daniel ...

When I met him, his left eyelid drooped slightly and his eyes appeared "out of sync" with one another. This gave him a dreamy, unfocused look. I gave him an exercise designed to lift his left eyelid and within about six months, his eyelids appeared the same. Also, lots of eye coordination and tracking exercises have made his eyes into more of a team, and now, when he looks at anything, he's focused and "right there". The difference is very noticeable.

Also, just a few months ago, Daniel ran into an old friend who happens to be an Optician. He explained enthusiastically about all he experienced and all that had improved for him in the past year or more. He was met with the same response from his old friend that I had received all those years ago, with the statement, "But the Bates stuff doesn't work. There's no science to back it up."

Daniel's response was, again, much like mine; "But here I am! You know how visually impaired I was before, and now I can see, man. That's proof enough for me!"

* * *

I am hoping that a doctor or scientist would like to come forward and study Daniel and others like him, comparing prior results with results today.

Some people call me naive, but I just can't help believing that we are all on the same page, really … that at the very heart of it, we all want health and the clearest, most natural vision possible for everyone. There is just too much evidence that so many of the natural principles work to continue to ignore them completely.

One very dependable fact is that if we do nothing to help ourselves, nothing will happen.

There are so many variables; practices that work for some people and don't work for others, situations where glasses are the best seeing solution and others where they are not, and so many circumstances in between.

In these times when cures are being discovered for conditions that used to be untreatable, most of us are ready to believe that nothing is hopeless, and there's always a possibility of recovery.

Isn't this something we want to know more about? Rather than study only visual illness, we could find ways of pointing back towards wellness. There are plenty of models out there of people who have improved their vision and many of them are quite anxious to talk about it to those who will listen!

As people open their minds to the possibility of good news, we can blow the old myths apart and learn a lot in the bargain.

CHAPTER FIVE

Sacred Territory

"The eye is the lamp of the body. When the eye is sound, the whole body will be filled with light."
— *Jesus of Nazareth*

Unquestionably, our eyes are key to our connection with one another. Messages from our eyes can be transmitted across a room, or from the driver of one car to another, instantly, and these messages are tremendously powerful. The light being transmitted is a part of the eyes' expression and is sent and received by most people without even considering the implications of this amazingly strong form of communication.

We have all sent messages of love, appreciation, sympathy, understanding, fear, anger and more, in a split second, simply through our eyes. How many of us can still recall that first "look of love" from someone we cherish, or a furtive glance that spoke volumes to us, even decades ago?

Regardless of the message, there is potential for a very strong impact.

Working with our eyesight can lift a veil for us that leads to whole new levels of awareness in our everyday living. We can become wiser, gentler, more courageous, more conscious, just more of who we really are when our eyes are working at their best configuration. With lenses removed, our eyes (the only parts of our bodies where light enters), become receptors to the full spectrum of light, and light is wisdom in its purest form.

As we make our entrance into this life, almost all of us have extremely good eyesight. Small children can see minute detail when examining something closely, and they also quickly develop the ability to see well far into the distance. They tend to see with wonder, with hearts and minds open to the new possibilities coming to them through their eyes. As darkness comes, children are ready to release and relax completely into a sleep that is deep and restorative, so that they can begin the next day with eyes that are refreshed and eager.

Somewhere between childhood and adulthood, we lose our ability to see with that kind of wonderful clarity. For many, the first loss of vision began just as a stressful episode was playing out in the outer world; loss of a parent, a move to a new home, divorce, arguments, bullies, and many other factors often stress a visually sensitive child into a state of blur.

With some understanding, blurry vision can be treated just like any other *temporary* problem, like influenza or an ear infection; a condition of weakness in the body that will pass, and meanwhile requires a little extra attention and tender loving care.

Unfortunately, many of us haven't known how to deal with the problem. I hear stories something like this from clients all the time:

"My vision blurred in sixth grade. I had my eyes examined and got glasses. Then, in eighth grade I needed stronger glasses, and then at the end of high school, my prescription got stronger again and I had astigmatism as well, and now, in middle age I'm wearing bifocal lenses because I can't see clearly at any distance and my Optometrist saw the beginning of a cataract, and ..."

... and on it goes.

It helps to consider the emotional and physical factors that might be contributing to the blurry vision, so that people can understand and cooperate in their own healing.

My own experience in middle age attests to the emotional factors. As I continued to work on improving my ability to see things up close, moving my focal point forward, there were times where I felt very uncomfortable with the process, even to the point where sometimes I would cry for no apparent reason.

Now I realize that I had begun to "push things away" from myself, by having a "blur zone" up close to me. Over the first two years, as I worked more diligently with my eyesight, I became more comfortable with having things close to me, and I addressed some of my "up close" needs; needs around intimacy and dreams I wanted to fulfill and claim, or re-claim, for my life. As things became clearer in my close visual field, my emotional needs also became clearer and it was much easier for me to understand and take action on these wishes.

My daughter had the opposite discomfort. She was uncomfortable with looking/seeing into the distance, and as her vision improved, we gently coaxed her out of this feeling.

Almost without exception, (and there have been a few exceptions), when I ask a client what was going on in their lives when they got that first pair of lenses for myopia, the answer is that there was tension and stress present. It seems as though they were unconsciously trying to make their personal world smaller and safer.

Without understanding the strong connection between weakened eyesight and stress, well-meaning parents take the child to a well-meaning Optometrist who measures the refractive error and prescribes glasses. Rooted in the onset of myopia is the fear of distance seeing and nothing has changed with the addition of lenses; the fear remains.

Now, the child must maintain this level of myopia in order to see through his new glasses. Chances of improvement have just been removed!

The adults involved in this very common scenario are doing what they think is best, for the most part because they are not aware that any alternative exists.

Let's imagine a situation where the response is different:

A child moves to a new neighbourhood where she feels very much out of place and alone. She is uncomfortable, looking around the schoolyard at all the unfamiliar faces and walking around an unfamiliar neighbourhood. She goes home and sits in her room, reading by the hour, escaping into her favourite books, where she feels much more comfortable, emotionally. It soon becomes obvious to her new teacher that she is having difficulty seeing the work at the front of the room.

Imagine that her parents and teachers realize that this early stage of near-sightedness could be a sign of stress. She is encouraged to talk about her uncomfortable feelings and not hide away all the time, reading. With some gentle guidance and attention, she finds new enjoyable activities within her small circle, that relax and rejuvenate her eyesight; activities like playing catch with a parent or friend, or fetch with a willing dog, or visiting beautiful new parks or the zoo. In this way, she comes to see some parts of her new life as non-threatening, and her body/being/eyes begin to relax again.

An understanding teacher can introduce her to activities at school that encourage her to look outward, like painting pictures of distant scenery or objects, or kite-flying, or bean-bag toss. There is bound to be a child who is interested in the same activities and the teacher can put these children together for mutual benefit and fun. Soon, she "fits in" and begins to feel more comfortable and secure where she is, in the present moment. Books become the exciting diversion they were meant to be, rather than her escape from "real life".

There are certainly some specific vision practices that can help stressed eyes to relax and heal and an understanding adult could teach her these, and help her to understand how to use her eyes in ways that keep them healthy.

On the other hand, if she is prescribed glasses she must maintain the same refractive error in order to continue to see through them.

I'm repeating myself because it's critical that we comprehend the above statement. Bates proved over and over again in his observations that vision is dynamic; we might see better in the morning after a good night's sleep, worse when we are in a rush, better when we are excited about the day, worse when we have an examination to write. In other words, our clarity of seeing changes often!

If we go to the Optometrist and are measured at a particular moment in time, and then fitted with prescription lenses based on those results, the implication here is that our blurry vision will not change; that we will continue to see in the same impaired way all day long and in all situations. This is simply not true.

As Bates discovered, behind our glasses dynamic vision slows or stops and our eyes become more and more dependent as they weaken. Moreover, as in the case with our young friend, no one has helped her to work with the underlying stressors in her life and she retreats from her new world, rather than experience the empowerment of learning to embrace her new challenges.

Which approach supports growth, independence, understanding and most importantly, overall health?

Everyone's story is different but the commonality is that stress is often the underlying factor. The earlier in life we learn to address and even embrace stress for the learning that it brings, the better.

Not everyone who becomes myopic does so because of emotional factors. Sometimes it is just what Bates identified; mental and physical strain. School and studies or staring at computers just for fun, or doing any kind of "near work" for long periods can cause us to lose flexibility in our eyes and lose distance vision.

There are so many simple ways to care for the eyes while learning and studying. The paradox is that the more relaxed our eyes are while we are learning, the more easily we learn and remember things. We simply don't learn as well or remember as well when our systems are stressed and tense, and of course, this is an unhealthy and unhappy way to conduct our school or professional lives, anyway.

Healthy habits are just as easily formed as unhealthy ones! Bates was quoted as saying, "People have just as much time to use their eyes correctly as incorrectly."

We can always look for another, healthier route to take. Switching on the television, it would appear that North Americans love to exist on diets of hamburgers, factory prepared food from our freezers, and lots of beer! But we know that this is not the stuff healthy bodies are made of, and more and more of us are doing our own investigating and making the healthiest, even if not the most convenient, choices.

Hallelujah for ourselves and for our children, as we support organic farmers, turn away from heavily meat-based or chemical-laden diets, drink more pure water, and detoxify and energize our bodies. In doing all of those things, of course, we support and nourish our eyes, the most nutritionally demanding parts of us.

I can remember playing "blind man's bluff" as a child, and the great relief and exhilaration I would feel when my blindfold came off! That's a game that teaches us to trust, for sure, as we are blindfolded by friends and led around; we have to trust that those leading us will not bring us to harm. But wow, when our eyes are open and the "lights are back on" we certainly learn to appreciate the sense of seeing. In fact, most people rank vision No. 1 as the capacity they would most dislike losing ... and yet, what precautions do we take (and do we know how to take) to preserve this wonderful sense?

Collectively, we have been duped. We are reminded to floss our teeth, moisturize our skin, wash our hair regularly, eat fibre for good digestion, and keep clean physically to avoid germs — all measures to guard our health, and yet, if public education is any indication, our eyes require no preventative measures to keep them healthy; just prescription glasses when they weaken and fail us.

But, please, who is failing whom? What are we doing to protect our vision and to teach our children to do the same?

Eyes, I would like to submit, are precious, and eyesight is, yes, sacred. We need to wake up, educate ourselves, and take care of our eyes and our vision. Eyesight links us to one another and to the world we live in. Over 90% of the information we take in over our lifetimes enters through our eyes. What could be more important?

Eyes that meet another's can foster love, trust and understanding, and show us the soul that shines behind those eyes we are meeting. This is sacred space; an intimate connection ... eyes shining back and forth at each other, emitting many energetic signals.

Close your eyes for 30 seconds. Is this not just the most precious commodity you have?

Everything changes when we improve, protect, and love our eyes, and everything shifts for the better when we can truly see.

As always, education is the liberator. Once we really understand the causes of our visual woes, we are on our way to correcting them. Always, though, eyes should be treated with a sense of reverence, because truly, they are the gateway to the path of light in the body and to a glimpse of the soul who resides there.

"Beauty is not in the clothes worn, the figure we carry, or the way we wear our hair. Beauty is seen in the eyes, because that is the doorway to our hearts, the place where love resides."
— Audrey Hepburn

The Sacred Practice of Palming

The practice of palming is the cornerstone of any Vision Improvement program. Because we know that weakened vision is a result of tension in the eyes, palming is the best way of reducing or eliminating that tension.

Before I explain why I consider this practice to be sacred, here's how it's done:

To palm your eyes, rub your hands together, until they are warm and full of energy. "Cup" them into the shape you would use to catch water and then place them over your closed eyes, with the heels of your hands on your cheek bones, and your fingertips overlapped and resting on your forehead ... there is no pressure on your eyes whatsoever, and as you breathe and relax, a "pocket" of warm, energetic air is created between your palms and your eyes.

Rest, rest, rest, as you focus inward, on the path of your breathing, and observe the darkness intensifying as you relax more and more. You can use this time to visualize something that gives you pleasure: a flower, a beloved pet, or some beautiful object. Place this focal point at a distance that normally challenges you and notice that as you imagine it, even at this challenging distance, you can see the shape and the object with perfect clarity and ease. Enjoy this, as you deepen your relaxation, both in your eyes and body.

When you are ready to open your eyes, first, take away your hands but leave your eyes closed for a minute or two as you adjust to the light. Then, when you open your eyes, blink 30 times or more and feel the stimulation of the blinking as you go back into "real" seeing.

That was easy and relaxing, yes? We know that the rods and cones — the cells on our retinas that are responsible for detail and colour — can only relax when in deep darkness, and so palming is the way to give our eyes some rest as we go through our long and busy days.

While we palm, those retinal cells get a full stretch in the darkness, as they are light sensors, and then close up more as we come back to the light. This gives them some exercise and stimulation as well as rest and the whole practice only need take five minutes or less.

Through palming, the retinal cells gradually become stronger in their ability to see detail and they handle light more efficiently. So, eyes become less light sensitive over time and they become better able to see contrast.

William Bates proved that when our eyes are relaxed, our bodies relax and vice-versa. So it's impossible to be completely physically relaxed with tense eyes.

Through the practice of palming combined with deep breathing, we coax our eyes, bodies and mental faculties into deeper and deeper relaxation. I consider this practice sacred because it takes us deep inside ourselves; deeper, I believe, than a regular meditation practice with eyes either open or closed, because, again, our eyes must be a part of the relaxation, and the blackness of palming gets us into this fully relaxed state.

The paradox of the eyes is that they make far better use of the light after spending time in darkness. So, when we sit and relax and palm and breathe deeply, we create a sacred space within ourselves where healing can occur.

Our hands are important players in the palming ritual. Our hands carry energy; we all know this either consciously or unconsciously. Think of all the different kinds of handshakes you've experienced. The old saying that you can tell a lot about a person by their handshake (or just by holding their hand for a minute) is very true. In the healing modality of Reiki, chi, or energy, is passed through the practitioner's hands into the body of the receiver, for healing. In palming with our own hands over our eyes, we are channeling our body energy towards healing our eyes.

Arms and hands are the extensions of our hearts. We reach out to touch and love and caress because of the impulse that originates in our hearts. I always ask my clients to breathe in deeply, feeling their heart and chest area fill with air, and then on the exhale, imagine directing this warm "chi" or energy from their hearts, down through their arms, into their hands and then into their eyes for healing.

I call this a "healing circle" created by our body posture. Our eyes have seen many things in our lifetimes that were difficult to look at, and taking time to send loving energy into our eyes encourages them to relax again and appreciate what they are seeing in the present moment.

Often, I notice a guardedness in people's looking that can be replaced by the loving energy channeled through palming in this way. Completely relaxed eyes sparkle and shine and engage directly with others ... and we can restore this kind of vibrance, courage and presence through a daily palming practice.

I suggest to people that they palm first thing in the morning, to start their day with refreshed eyes, again around lunchtime, again around dinnertime, and before bed, so that they go to sleep with eyes relaxed. Keeping your bedroom very dark is important too, so that your whole visual system can rest fully, in the blackness.

How We Got Here

If we take a minute to look at things historically, we can begin to understand how we got to this place, where so many eyes are ailing. It wasn't always this way.

Way back in the 1400's, in Mainz, Germany, Johannes Guggenheim invented the printing press, which certainly revolutionized the world by creating a way for us to mass produce printed books and papers. By the end of the 19th century, the printing press was in common use worldwide.

Also, by the early 20th century, thanks to the pioneering work of several inventors like Davy, Swan and Edison, we ended up with the mass production of the electric light bulb to light up our homes at any time of day.

Combine these two inventions — printed books and newspapers available for purchase and houses that could be bright as daylight after sundown, and this is the place where life began to change irrevocably for our eyes. (Of course, people had experienced vision problems before that time in history, but the situation grew increasingly worse into the 20th century and beyond.)

Through this time, all over the world, eyeglasses in various forms were being developed and by the early 20th century, the field of Optics was being recognized and the production of "spectacles" for common use began. More and more effort was directed towards developing specific glasses for the use of specific eyes, displaying myopia or presbyopia, or both, and/or astigmatism in one or both eyes.

And so, as we were staying up late and reading or sewing under electric lights, extending our days by many hours, our eyes were working very hard to keep up. Eventually, visual problems began to occur, but voila! — a solution had emerged in the form of eyeglasses.

These lenses appear miraculous and really, they are wonderful for giving us the ability to see again. As the Optometrist said to me in 1995, "Just get these glasses and wear them."

And that's what we've all been doing for a century or so. But how is it working out for us?

William Bates was able to see where we were headed more than 80 years ago, and he proposed that we step back and look at this again, in a different way.

If we want our eyes to stay up late and work longer hours for us, all the time, what we must do for our eyes is give them more rest. They need darkness to rest and that's what palming is all about.

We are also at a point in history where we have prized hard work and education above all else, but we are learning now, in more areas than just visual, that we cannot place anything above our health.

CHAPTER SIX

Myopia, Astigmatism and Other Blurs

"Your imagination is your preview of life's coming attractions."
— Albert Einstein

To take the mystery out of the word myopia, let's remember that it simply means near-sightedness — the first word, *near*, describing where we see best. So a near-sighted (myopic) person can "see-well-near" but has trouble seeing further away, into the distance.

Before we go any further, let's understand what the prescription means. If you don't happen to have a copy of your prescription, your Optometrist can supply it to you.

Here's an example of a prescription for near-sightedness or myopia. Often myopic people have astigmatism numbers as well and we'll discuss those in a minute.

Decoding A Prescription

	Sphere (Power)
OD (right eye)	-2.50 (diopters)
OS (left eye)	-3.25 (diopters)

Diopters are the units of measure that define how strong your glasses need to be to bring you to 20/20 seeing. (20/20 meaning the ability to read a letter that is one-inch high from a distance of 20 feet)

The higher the number of diopters, the stronger the lenses. So, if your glasses are -2.00 or so, you have a mild correction, -5.00 is a moderate correction, and -10.00 diopters, a strong correction. In many cases, as in the one illustrated above, each eye has been prescribed a different number of diopters to bring it to 20/20.

Normal eyes are flexible and very dynamic in the way that they operate. The extra-ocular muscles flex and relax, flex and relax, to see close and far, close and far, and this flexing creates healthy circulation and eyes that see clearly. For the myopic person, the muscles have remained "stuck" in flex mode.

Optometrists will describe the near-sighted or myopic person as having eyeballs that are elongated from front to back. Some professionals describe them as "football shaped".

When light enters an eyeball that is unnaturally long, the image is dropped in front of the retina, rather than squarely in the centre, where clear seeing occurs. And so, the near-sighted person begins to squint, unconsciously trying to somehow move forward to where that image is dangling in front of his retina. (Excessive squinting, while it might help sometimes in the short-term, actually increases the whole problem because it makes the eye muscles more tense.)

One question that is rarely voiced or discussed: If, for example, an 8-year-old child is diagnosed with an elongated eyeball and prescribed glasses, what was going on when this child was seven years old — last year, when he could see just fine? What happened?

The answer to that question is obvious. Somewhere in the past year, that child's eyeball has changed shape. At this point, some professionals will allude to the possible cause being visual stress or stress of some sort, but they generally suggest only one remedy. Prescription glasses.

If Bates was correct, the newly tensed eye muscles are causing the problem, and those muscles can be re-trained to relax when seeing clearly. Deep relaxation frees the eyeball so that it can resume its natural shape and work dynamically again. Then the image will drop squarely on the retina and the problem will truly be corrected!

Naturally. Simply. And the earlier in life, the better, which is why I'm so passionate about getting this message to parents, and through them, to children.

Dr. Bates noted over and over again that once prescription glasses are introduced, the muscle dynamics and shifting shape of the eyeball, just stops. The glasses are doing the work now and we continue to need them in order to see, so we buy and buy and buy glasses, even being coaxed into selecting "fashionable" ones to make ourselves feel better about wearing them all day.

Unless, perhaps, someone intervenes before all this happens, and teaches the person how to "unlock" those frozen muscles and create a state of dynamic tension again, so that their eyes are then free to see well, as they did a month or a year previously.

Natural Vision Improvement methods point in a whole new direction that can serve to open up new possibilities for individuals whose visual world is shrinking, while their visual health is deteriorating.

Factors that sometimes complicate the near-sighted situation are feelings of fear, mistrust and tension that may have been developed with seeing. Near-sighted people sometimes have difficulty trusting what they see or perceive, and so this creates an on-going sense of tension and fear, which creates more tension and blur, and on it goes ...

A good Vision Educator can help the myope to discern the "how" of their looking so that they can perceive images in a fresh way, in the present, rather than looking through a "fear lens" based on the past. Whether the past stressful situation occurred last week or twenty years ago, the remedy is the same; we must release the eyes, so that we don't adopt a permanent "deer in the headlights" way of looking at life.

Obviously, though, if someone has been holding their eyes in a state of tension for twenty years, it will probably take longer to relax those eyes than if the tension has only been a reality for one year. Again, that's the reason why childhood is the best time to deflect the problems of near-sight. New habits tend to be easier to break, but all habits of seeing can be changed and improved.

When I meet a client whose vision correction is over -10 diopters, without exception in my experience so far, there has been a situation of abuse and/or trauma in the past; either emotional or physical, or both. An abused or bullied child is often so frozen in fear that he/she is completely afraid to see, whether aware of that or not. It's just more comfortable to be in a blurry world than to look right into the eyes of your abuser or an abusive situation.

When this child is given stronger and stronger lenses over time, the real problem has not been addressed, and so it cripples the eyes' ability to see and function in a healthy way. Our eyes and brain try to work completely in sync, and it is the brain that commands the eyes' response. Should the brain make the decision to create blur for any reason, it could send out the corresponding commands to the eyes, holding them in the right state of tension which could block out the world that the child doesn't want to see.

So, on the psychological level, myopia can be a method of retracting, or pulling away, from vision.

It's a way of expressing, "I can see things up close to me, in my comfort zone, but things at a distance can be threatening, so I've decided to blur them out. What I can't see, can't hurt me." This is not always the case, as sometimes myopia is a simple result of too much reading or computer work, but in my experience, fear and tension usually work together to cause the blurry state.

Of course, the prescription glasses bring the child's eyes right back to clarity, but what if this is hugely uncomfortable at some level, and none of the underlying causes have been noticed or considered? The eyes have to weaken quickly, or the child must detach emotionally from what is being seen so clearly, or both.

Why not at least try the natural route first? Nothing to lose and everything to gain. In many cases, people don't realize they have a choice, which is why this book and others like it exists.

When we are "stuck" in a fearful place, over time, we become critical of ourselves and others (the fear makes us watchful), and often judgmental. Fear can stop us from engaging with others and with life even after the actual threat that might have been experienced long ago, is past.

Myopic people often become extremely detail-oriented and linear in their thinking, and of course, these patterns can be very limiting. I've worked with people with strong prescriptions who often feel unsupported, and even despairing. Depression often lifts as the veil of lenses and blur is lifted and light goes into the body again, undeterred. Easy does it, however — and vision, when improved naturally, is a gradual return to clarity; not a "quick fix".

Spiritually, since the lens used for myopia creates a virtual image, there can often be a feeling of "unreality" accompanying this kind of seeing. The lens focuses light on the macula alone, and deprives the retina of a more equal distribution of light. As more of the retina is stimulated with light through NVI practices, more of the brain is involved in seeing.

Have you ever noticed how people smile more on that first brilliant sunshiny spring day? That's the way it feels to be freed of lenses and to, once again, experience the distribution of light evenly over the retinal cells, and down into the body.

"Hallelujah! The light has returned to my being!" Literally, that's the feeling and it's worth working for.

Improving vision naturally and gradually — addressing any issues as they come up as we reverse the process of visual deterioration — is akin to throwing off shackles that are completely outdated and setting ourselves free to see happily again. That's so much closer to the way we were meant to live, and to see.

So many people are deprived of the joyful seeing that is their birthright. In North America alone, over *seventy million people* are nearsighted and the numbers are growing!

Astigmatism

Astigmatism (which tends to accompany myopia) is a distortion in one plane of vision — vertical, horizontal or anywhere in between. It appears to be the result of a misshapen area in the cornea, which causes problems with seeing on one plane of vision, thus creating even more blur.

For anyone with astigmatism in one or both eyes there will be two more categories on the prescription; Cylinder and Axis. The cylinder number identifies the amount of extra power needed in one area, and the axis number gives the location of the astigmatic area in the eye. And again, the right and left eye are often different.

	Sphere	Cylinder	Axis
OD (right)	-2.50	-0.25	042
OS (left)	-3.25	-0.50	174

For a very simple example, if you have a vertical (90) astigmatism, that would mean that when you look at something in the vertical plane (like a straight flag pole, for example), there would appear to be a bit of a bump in it. Astigmatism often accompanies myopia and prescriptions reflect this; that is, prescription lenses make an adjustment so that little bump is gone when you look at the flagpole with your glasses on.

Mainstream thinking appears to be that once someone shows up in the Optometrist's chair and demonstrates an astigmatism on examination, they need correction for it. However, if we accept what Bates was teaching; that seeing and our way of seeing is dynamic and changing all the time, then isn't it just possible that if I'm stressed or upset or exhausted, I might develop an astigmatism for a time that might disappear later when things settle down? Of course it's possible. Our bodies are regenerating at an alarmingly fast rate and anything can heal or change.

Joy Thompson

Think about this; if I get my prescription filled with the astigmatism correction, I *must maintain the astigmatism* in order to see through the glasses! So now, when I take off those glasses that make my vision perfect, there's all that blur and that darn bump in the flagpole again and any other vertical lines look weird, and I get quite uncomfortable (of course) and have to go find my glasses in order to see "normally". See where this is going? Towards more and more dependency on glasses and the impossibility of healing that astigmatic condition, or the near-sightedness that goes with it.

I had a personal experience with what seemed like astigmatism when my son was seventeen. He was very badly injured in an accident and we were both terrified as I raced my car to the hospital. On arrival, I was as close to hysterics as I've ever been, looking at my son who was so badly hurt and in such pain.

The authorities at the hospital said that before they could take my son in and care for him, I had to fill out a form. As I picked up the pen and looked at the form, the writing was a complete blur; I couldn't read any of it, even though, of course, I normally had excellent vision.

As I looked at the page, all the lines on it were bumpy and crooked as well as the letters all being blurry. I remember thinking, "Wow, I have about 100 astigmatisms going on here." The nurse (thankfully) sat me down and filled out the form for me as I dictated the answers as best I could.

My son was taken into Emergency and cared for very well, and late that night, we went home exhausted. Realizing he was comfortably asleep, I finally settled in and got some restorative sleep myself. The next morning, I picked up a newspaper to see whether my eyes had actually recovered, and I could see again, perfectly — no bumps, distortions or blur anymore.

Sometimes I think that I've been provided with so many visual experiences, just so I can develop a healthy perspective in working with visual challenges. I know that if someone in the hospital that night had examined my eyes, I would have been assessed as badly needing vision correction, even though, within 24 hours, all was well again. My eyes were in trauma for a time, as was the rest of my body, but given the right conditions, the trauma and all its manifestations passed.

My experience is a dramatic example, but suppose someone is feeling a generalized worry or fear that causes a distortion in one plane of seeing for a time ... uncorrected, there is an opportunity for the condition to right itself naturally with a little patience and knowledge.

It appears that common thinking is that once someone has astigmatism it is likely to stay there. At least, there seems to be no concern about it remaining until the next examination occurs and as mentioned, as long as the glasses are used, that's very likely going to be true.

Eyes that Spoke Volumes

When I was a little girl, I distinctly remember sitting with my Dad one time on a very hot summer day. His face was wet and sweating and he decided to remove his glasses for a few minutes. It was, really, the first time I ever saw his eyes. He wore thick, "coke bottle" glasses and had since shortly after immigrating to Canada when he was eleven years of age.

His mother had died of cancer and his father, suffering from a completely broken heart since her loss, decided to take his young son and get on a boat that set sail from Liverpool, England, to start what he hoped would be a happier new life, in Canada.

And so, my Dad lost his mother, his home, his country, close friends, neighbourhood, school, his dog, his soccer team — everything he held dear, in one tragic year. Already myopic, his development of highly impaired vision followed rapidly. At the tender age of eleven, he went to work in an Ontario factory alongside my Grandfather, and the two tried to make their way in a strange, and sometimes hostile, new place.

On that day three decades later, when he removed his glasses and looked at me, I don't know what he saw through his myopic eyes, but I was forever changed, looking into his unprotected eyes that first time. I noticed how tender and vulnerable his eyes looked, such a soft blue — and I perceived a sadness and yearning there as well.

The skin behind his glasses was much paler than the rest of his face, from having worn lenses all the time. I also remember noticing markings in his eyes that were whimsical white swirls in his blue irises. I could feel his highly emotional nature and I could almost hear that frightened young boy's cries for help and security. It was all still there, in those lovely soft eyes and the emotion I felt in response surprised me, and touched me very deeply.

After that, I always felt that I knew a secret about my Father that he was possibly not aware of himself. As a Vision Educator, I know now that so much fear and sadness within held him back from activities and expansion beyond the secure world that he had finally managed to create for himself.

Part of the reason I am so committed to my work is because I know that my Dad would have welcomed the opportunity to allow healing in and to expand his visual field. He was never offered that chance, but would approve of me helping others in this way; helping them to liberate themselves from blurry vision, which is so often the result of stress and fatigue.

Eye Massage

The term "eye massage" is a little misleading, because of course we don't massage the eyes, but rather the soft area around the eye socket, which is where those extra-ocular muscles live.

Just like any other muscles, these tiny ones respond beautifully to touch; the stimulation increases circulation to the area and encourages the muscles to relax. I massage my eyes once each day at least, and my clients do as well. Everybody reports back to me that this simple practice feels so good!

Begin at the inner corners, above your eyes. I use my thumbs. Press upwards, away from the eyeball (no pressure is ever placed on the eyeball itself) towards the eyebrow bone. Breathe deeply and relax as you gently stimulate the area. Then slowly move towards the outside of the eye, stopping to press and release or massage in circles, within the hollow above your eye.

Gently, gently, does it.

Once you've completed massaging the area above your eye, using pointer fingers and again, gentle pressure, massage from the inner corner of your eye to the outer corner, below the eye — in the hollow between your eye and your cheekbone, massaging down toward the bone, away from the eye.

To complete, take your thumb and pointer finger and massage those little bumps in the inside corners of your eyes (often we do this naturally for eye strain). This is the final step in eye massage.

If done on a regular basis, the practice of eye massage encourages the eye muscles to relax and also increases circulation to the whole area, making it more alive and full of energy.

Complete by palming and then blinking. Thank your eyes for all the work they do!

Blinking

Blinking stimulates the muscles that encircle our eyes; enlivens them by increasing circulation and loosening them up. Sometimes those muscles have been tight for many years and blinking is a quick way of releasing tension in our eyes and stimulating them.

So, as you come out of your palming sessions, always take your hands away from your closed eyes and allow them to adjust to the light coming through your eyelids. Then blink many times — at least 30, to stimulate your eyes with light and awaken those muscles. Feels good!

Near-sighted people tend to stare unblinkingly at books or screens and are often completely unaware of this habit. Just placing a sign on your computer screen — as well as a few reminders around the house — can help you to get back to the healthy habit of blinking about once every three seconds.

Of course, blinking also helps to lubricate the cornea with one of the most sophisticated protective substances in the world; human tears. Natural chemical protection is furnished by the tear glands, located just above the eyes. Every time we blink, we lubricate and disinfect the surface of our eyes with this incredibly beneficial liquid.

Such lubrication can make a huge difference in protecting our eyes from viruses and pollutants in the air, as well as keeping the eye muscles in that happy state of dynamic relaxation while they are working.

Swaying

Swaying back and forth with eyes open and relaxed is an extremely soothing activity for the eyes as well as the body. Watch a new mother holding her baby as she gently, automatically, sways back and forth. That movement is soothing them both.

When I do my swaying, I like to have some soft, slow music on. If I sway for the 3 minutes it takes to play the song, I'll be in a lovely, relaxed state when the music is finished. And it's all so easy. Some people like to sway for longer, but even just the three minutes' time is very valuable.

As we sway, our eyes will be coaxed to stop "trying to see" as the blurry world passes us by. Place your feet about shoulder-width apart, let your arms swing loosely as you turn back and forth, lifting your back heel to allow a half-turn to each side. Keep your head and neck in line with your spine as you move.

Notice the blur that's created as you swing. Notice that as you turn to the right, the whole world seems to move to the left, and vice-versa. Develop a lovely, deep rhythm to your breathing as you sway back and forth. Allow the blur to just be there, and feel the support of your body as you sway.

You can vary this practice by looking at your thumb as you sway back and forth; noticing the stable image of your thumb with the blurred background behind. Breathe rhythmically, again "tuning in" to the stability of your body, the steadiness of the thumb image, and the gentleness of the blur you can see in the background.

For the same reason that swaying benefits and relaxes our eyes and bodies, swinging on swings or in hammocks, rocking in rocking chairs, or just watching the world fly by as a passenger in a car or train are all activities that can allow us to let go, relax and release.

When I work with children, they are often delighted to learn that the "homework" I'm assigning is to go to the park and swing on the swings! Some kids have forgotten the joy and abandon that can be felt in that kind of rhythmic motion, when their bodies and eyes have let go and relaxed into it.

CHAPTER SEVEN

Far-sightedness

"What can it profit a man to gain the whole world and to come to his property with ... bifocals?"
— John Steinbeck

Far-sightedness, or what is called "hyperopia" in younger folks and "presbyopia" when it comes along in middle age, is the condition of being able to see well into the distance but seeing blur up close. If someone is prescribed glasses for far-sightedness, it will be in the form of "plus lenses"; +1.00 diopter being a mild prescription and +4.00 or higher, a strong correction for far-sight.

Sheila

Sheila contacted me very recently, concerned about her reading vision and how she was hoping to improve it before embarking on some extended travel. Her goals were simple; just wanting to "unload" the reading glasses and sharpen her vision at all distances.

She had recently experienced a divorce but felt that the stress of that time was passed, and she easily focused on moving forward.

Over the next two months, Sheila and I met weekly. She was a pleasure to work with, performing her daily vision practices faithfully.

After two months, Sheila and I had achieved all of the goals we had set when we began. Her right eye had strengthened and both eyes were performing beautifully together. She no longer experienced eye strain or got headaches when working at her computer or reading, and she was completely glasses-free. She also noticed that she was no longer light-sensitive and used her sunglasses only when the sun's glare was very bright. Also, her night vision was strong and she commented that colours seemed more vibrant.

Sometimes, the work that I do is very simple and my collaboration with Sheila was definitely one of those times. She knew herself well, and there were no psychological or emotional blocks in her way. She was absolutely ready to strengthen her eyes and move towards a clear future, and she has done just that.

As presbyopia comes along in middle age, it is considered by many to be "normal" and "part of the aging process". It is more a result of neglect than age. If we haven't stimulated a body part in 20 or 30 or 40 or 50 years, it is likely to become weak!

Can our focusing mechanism be strengthened? The answer is a resounding, "yes"! and once we reclaim our ability to see "up close" again, many things can change in our physical, intellectual, psychological and spiritual world, to add to the huge benefit of improved eyesight.

Hyperopic children are sometimes slower to learn to read and more active generally, often being labeled as "hyperactive" when actually, it is their focusing mechanism that is stressed and causing them to want to look away, at something further into the distance (and therefore easier to look at). That was my story so I know it well.

From the hyperopic child's point of view, he may be sitting at his desk in school, trying to read the assigned pages. He's fine for a while, but then, without him even realizing it, his eye muscles are tired of holding the flex, and when he looks up and gazes across the room, he feels more comfortable.

He thinks, "Maybe I'll just sharpen my pencil and then come back and read" — and off he goes, but on the way back, he passes by his friend's desk and his friend makes a face at him and the two start giggling and .... well, this is how it goes, and such a child can easily be labeled a troublemaker (really, who needs a sharp pencil to read, anyway?).

But of course, the pencil and the friend aren't the issue, necessarily. It's the underlying (and unconscious) need to move away from the stress of holding focus at the near point.

A child like this, by the way, could be taken to an Optometrist and evaluated as having good vision, because of course he can see all that he needs to for the exam. It is the maintaining of close focus that is a challenge for this child.

Rather than discipline or try to control, in some way, a child like this, (as is often the case), we could help to re-train their eyes to see at close range, and also teach them, and all children, how to manage close work without causing eye strain. These practices can be taught within one interactive classroom lesson and simply reinforced with a few simple routines and the good examples of adults.

This might seem overly simplistic, but let's not underestimate the importance of having strong eyes. Eyes that can focus quickly at all different distances, hold that focus, work well with the light, see contrast, subtleties of colour and movement, and more, are key to learning with ease. These eyes rest deeply at night and are refreshed and all ready to go the next day! Healthy eyes and good eyesight are part of the pleasure of living and learning that should be enjoyed by every child.

In middle-age, often eye muscles begin to show weakness — again, because we have not been caring for them properly for decades. This does not have to mean a new pair of bi-focals, or stronger and stronger reading glasses for life. Shiela and I are evidence of that as are hundreds more people over 40 who have maintained or improved the fitness of their visual systems and do not require glasses in order to see up close.

In my experience, middle-age comes with a number of emotional/spiritual challenges as well and the link to the way we are seeing things is often quite obvious.

As we enter mid-life, many of us become concerned with "far-sighted" types of issues. It is in these years that we often re-evaluate our lives with questions like:

"What have I still not accomplished that I want to give attention to at this stage in my life?"

"What's most important to me?"

"Have I fulfilled my goals?"

"Am I ready to take a new direction?"

"Am I satisfied with my accomplishments/relationships/level of self-knowledge?"

These are examples of the deeper questions of life and as we gaze off into the horizon, we may want to contemplate where we've been and where we are going. If it all looks clear in the distance (i.e.. we know what we want and where we'd like to be) but fuzzy up close (the details of how to get there are overwhelming), this is when some people give up and make statements like, "I'm too old now". "Guess I won't get there — I'll just be content with where I am and make the best of it" — but these are strategies for coping with lost dreams.

What might certainly be preferable would be to set a whole new challenge; one that is achievable and exciting. Now, perhaps we're ready to see those details and make a whole new plan! This requires us being able to see "up close" — very close and personal — and sort out where we are and where we want to go in the second half of life. Clearing and strengthening close eyesight can be the most wonderful tool for gaining insight, clarity and direction.

As "elders" in society we have much that we can contribute in the second half of our lives. There is more to life than gathering in coffee shops, playing golf, shopping in malls, and watching the news. All of these activities are fine in themselves, but not the sort of stuff for building a life around.

Ask any physician how often he sees retirees and finds them suffering from depression, illnesses, and lack of energy and drive and you'll learn that the numbers are high. Not long ago, taking the position of "elder" in the family or in society signified an exciting time where meaningful work could be done and knowledge imparted — not just empty time to be filled.

For me, improving my close vision in early middle age coincided with my passion to become a Vision Educator so it seemed like a "perfect fit" in so many ways ... but in continually working with my close vision I found I still had plenty to discover about myself. Unmet needs, passions and goals continue to surface, and it's been an interesting and eventful time.

Joan's Story

Joan was 56 when I met her. She's a beautiful, strong and very intelligent wife and mother and she had just arrived at a new threshold in her life. Her children were grown and living successfully on their own and her husband was about to retire from his professional life.

First on their agenda was a long-awaited trek through Europe that would last at least six months and take them through countries they had long dreamed of seeing. Joan was concerned because in the past few months her close vision was deteriorating quite rapidly, especially in her left eye, and she wasn't happy at the prospect of having to use glasses all the time for their extended vacation.

As we worked together and her vision began to improve, strong emotions surfaced for Joan. She realized that she was concerned with her husband being "up close and personal" all the time, once he was retired. She had always been very independent and was disconcerted about losing that independence suddenly. Also, she was more than a little worried about their relationship and how it would be with "all this togetherness"!

These were matters that weren't part of Joan's consciousness until her close vision began to improve and she realized these were issues needing attention.

Joan subsequently opened her concerns up to her husband who was having his own worries about his impending retirement, and the two were able to begin a whole new dialog. Once things were out in the open, they were able to come up with a plan for the future that made space for independence as well as a new creative cooperation between the two of them.

Joan continued to work on the physical exercises for her vision and within two months, she no longer required glasses for reading regular print. The next month, she left her reading glasses at home and headed off with her husband for the adventure of a lifetime. I still remember how her eyes sparkled the last time I saw her; all that was reflected there was pure excitement about what was right before her.

This is just another of many examples of how clearing vision can bring us joy and clarity in many areas of our lives. Some people don't experience the kind of emotions Joan was going through, but do clear their close vision anyway, with nothing in the way of that but deep relaxation and the right stimulation.

In every case I've worked with, people sense an enormous freedom in not requiring glasses for "up close" activities. I believe that some of that satisfaction comes from participating in their own healing; realizing that something can be done about their failing vision, and they can participate and make the changes necessary themselves!

The Sacred Practice of Sunning

The only other vision practice that I want to call "sacred" is the practice of sunning. In palming we bathe our eyes in darkness so that we can rest deeply, inside ourselves, in quiet, soothing space. In sunning, we call on the sun's magical rays to enlighten and enliven us; our eyes as well as our larger selves.

To "sun" your eyes, go outside and stand in the morning light or the light of late afternoon. Assume the stance you use for swaying as described in Chapter Six, and then close your eyes and turn them towards the sun. Sway gently back and forth, back and forth, keeping your head aligned with your spine as you twist gently to the right and then to the left. Breathe in deeply as you turn in one direction and exhale fully as you turn back to the other side.

As you breathe, enjoy the beautiful soothing sensations you feel as the sun touches your eyelids and the gentle light stimulates your eyes. Behind your closed lids, you will notice the very brightest space as where your closed eyes are facing the sun directly, and also the darkening as you turn to each side.

Turn back and forth, breathing deeply and slowly, about twenty times. You will feel your eyes and body relaxing more and more as you get comfortable with the movement. Next, turn your back to the sun and palm for about ten long, slow breaths.

Repeat the above one more time. The brightness of sunning, contrasted with the darkness of palming, stimulates your retinal cells — those cells responsible for discerning contrast and colour.

Do this practice on a daily basis, and over time, you will probably notice some of the benefits of this easy vision practice; you will be able to distinguish the contrast of light and dark more easily, colours appear more vibrant and the contrast of colours will appear more pronounced, you will be less light-sensitive, and your night vision will be clearer. Many people, myself included, simply feel better overall, physically as well as emotionally, just from incorporating this wonderful light routine into their days.

Make sure that after your final palming in the sunning routine, you take your hands away from closed eyes while they adjust again to the light, and practice lots of blinking before opening your eyes.

The sun is everything, isn't it? It is light and warmth and blessing and soothing and sweetness. Our eyes, when "well-sunned", as Bates described it, function healthfully and handle the light with ease.

Eye Crossing Exercise

To strengthen the muscles that help your eyes focus up close:

Stretch one arm out full-length and pop your thumb up. Cover your left eye and focus on the thumb with your right eye while you bring your thumb up as close to your nose as you can get it and still see it, (even if it's blurry). Now hold focus on the thumb for two long, slow breaths.

Next, repeat the practice, covering your right eye and doing the looking with your left eye.

Now, do the same practice looking with both eyes. Bring your thumb in as close to your nose as you can get it without it getting too fuzzy or doubling. Hold for two long, slow breaths. Finish by palming.

Jumping Focus

Stand outside or at your window and look off into the far distance, focusing on something in particular. Next, move your focus in to something closer, then something closer, something closer still, and then look at your thumb, placed directly in front of your nose.

(For example, when I do this exercise, I focus on a large tree on top of the hill in the distance, then on a chimney on a roof about a block away, then on my neighbour's gate, then my patio umbrella, and then my thumb.)

Make sure you're looking at something specific as you "jump" your eyes closer and closer. Then zoom way back out into the far distance and repeat.

Palm and breathe deeply to relax.

Accommodation Exercise

This exercise as well as the previous one help us to practice re-focusing quickly at different distances, an especially important skill for driving.

Extend one arm fully and pop your thumb up. Bring the other hand close to your nose — just a few inches away — and pop up the thumb directly in the line of sight of the distant thumb.

Look at front thumb, back thumb, front, back, and keep repeating very quickly. Work your eyes a little bit and then palm.

Break Time

When reading, sewing, working at the computer, or doing other close work, make a "30-minute rule" to keep your eyes from getting tired. Fatigue is a big enemy of healthy, clear vision.

After 25 minutes of close work, look into the distance and shift your eyes up, down, right, left, and diagonally, to give them a stretch. Palm and then do lots of blinking to rest and stimulate your eyes before going back to your work.

Visualization

When you are palming, visualize something up close and examine every minute detail. To keep my natural far-sightedness in check, I use different flowers for this exercise, and I imagine them so close to me that I can smell their fragrance, and then I trace my eyes around the petals and examine every nuance of colour and detail.

Our brain configures our eyes in exactly the same way when we are imagining something as when we actually are seeing it, so it behooves us to do this visualization, stimulating our brain/eyes/body to see up close again.

It's a good idea, while visualizing something up very close, to ask yourself how it feels to have something that close and to see it. It was easy for me at first, to imagine having a rose up close to my nose and enjoying it so much, but then, when I imagined different people up close to me, things changed.

Later on as I worked with my eyes, I found it interesting to explore how it felt to be "up close" in my imagination with someone who made me feel uncomfortable in the "real world". I realized that I felt squeamish in these cases, and that squeamishness kept me from really understanding what was going on in the present moment with them, because my discomfort was actually based on the past.

I discovered that no one was ever getting a fresh start with me! Visualizing and deep breathing took me to places in my imagination that were much more in the present — more relaxed and happy — and I learned gradually to see that way more and more in "real time". That was a very beneficial and personal side effect of improving my close vision.

If you are near-sighted, visualize something further away from you — anything that you enjoy seeing, like a beautiful tree or a rainbow, and feel yourself relaxing as you look far off. Practice that until it becomes a body habit to breathe and go into a state of relaxation while palming.

William Bates suggested that we imagine something black against a black background. I like to visualize a beautiful black horse running at night, imagining the sheen of his coat and the contours of his muscles, and his free-flowing mane and tail as he runs. It's a beautiful image which stands out surprisingly against the black background. Bates' premise was that the "black on black" visualization coupled with the darkness of palming, is especially relaxing.

Whatever you are visualizing, it's important you are imagining something that you can relax while seeing, because that is the key. We don't have to strain and "go out and get" the images with our eyes by doing anything. When we are relaxed, images just come to us and seeing is easy.

A lot of people have expressed to me that they "can't visualize", but anybody can. You don't have to be seeing the image of something as you would on a TV screen. It's enough just to be thinking about it. And the more you practice, the easier it gets.

CHAPTER EIGHT

Children's Vision

"The health of the eye seems to demand a horizon. We are never tired, so long as we can see far enough."
— *Ralph Waldo Emerson*

Emerson's quote certainly applies to children! Have you ever seen happy, active, well-seeing children who were easily tired? Ask their parents; they seem to go forever and the world is full of magic and enchantment for these kids.

Olivia's Story

This spring, I began working with a beautiful seven-year-old girl named Olivia. Her father had found me by searching the internet, and called me to discuss his daughter's prescription.

At the young age of 6, she had been fitted with a pair of glasses, complete with a correction for astigmatism, but then, one year later, she had been prescribed glasses that were double in strength, (-4 diopters in each eye) and her parents were baffled ... Why would such a young, healthy girl be losing her vision so quickly?

They were really shocked about her rapidly worsening near-sightedness and the Optometrist had no explanation for them, except to say something about her "growing too fast". They were mystified and concerned.

Working with Olivia has been such a delight for me, because she was eager to improve her vision and accepted the idea immediately. She listened to my explanations and instructions carefully, and then would just go off and integrate her vision practices into her daily routine — no problem.

I have to add that her parents have been wonderfully supportive. They were both present when I met with Olivia, so everybody understood the plan and all questions were answered at each session. Olivia's Mom helped her to create a schedule which they followed without fail. When we met, there were no excuses ... "Oh, we forgot for a few days", "We were too busy this week", "I wasn't feeling well so missed several days", etc. etc.

They just showed up every day despite their very busy schedule, colds or illness cropping up, etc. and did the Natural Vision practices! The whole family was committed. After 5 weeks like this, there was a noticeable improvement.

We all agreed that it was time for Olivia to be re-evaluated by an Optometrist, and I recommended one who would be cooperative and give Olivia a 20/40 prescription that would be much easier on her eyes and vision while we were working together. Olivia was anxious to see him, because her - 4.00 lenses were feeling too strong and seemed to be giving her headaches.

I am delighted to say that into her second month of Natural Vision Improvement practices, Olivia was back to wearing -2 lenses — back to half what she was wearing previously, and she only used them at school, when the board work was detailed and still blurry for her. She said the -2's felt just right, and the - 4's were rejected completely.

We continued to work with the practices and to meet weekly. By the last two weeks of school, Olivia was going without glasses completely! She said the board work was clear and she just "kept forgetting to put them on". (Yahoo!)

I suggested to Olivia that she keep her -2's with her, and then if she has a blurry moment, she can pull them out. So far, apparently, that hasn't been necessary. Now, in preparing for her summer vacation with family in Europe, she's packing her glasses but "doesn't expect to use them".

Olivia's parents have given her one of the greatest gifts a child can be given, in my opinion. Guiding her along and supporting her, they have helped her take her eyesight back and into her own hands (literally, because she palms a lot and loves it) and helped her unload those strong lenses at this early stage.

Olivia's a very lucky girl for two reasons: the persistence of her parents in finding another way, and their commitment to helping her reclaim the clear vision she'd had only a couple of years before. She'll never forget this experience, and her eyesight will likely be stronger and healthier for life.

A couple of very happy side-effects; Olivia's Mom did all the exercises with her daughter and after 3 months, she no longer needs her -2's, which she had been wearing for many years. She was tested and doesn't require glasses for driving anymore, so she is also glasses-free.

Olivia's Dad did the practices too, as well as a few extra I gave him for presbyopia. He had trouble reading and thought he would need reading/computer glasses soon. After the same three months, he is seeing fine now at all distances.

Thomas

I have another client who is in his 20's and started with me with a prescription of -13 in each eye. This is an extremely strong prescription for such a young man. When we began our work together, he was able to read just a few of the largest letters on my large eye chart when he was standing only 18 inches away from it. He began to wear lenses at age six and was wearing -4's, all the time, when he was very young, as he was growing and forming habits. He was in an abusive situation as a young lad, and there was a lot of fear involved in his daily life because he was keeping secrets, out of fear.

Now, at age 26, having faithfully worn glasses all these years (believing sincerely that this was the healthy thing to do for his eyesight), he has a strong dependency on these thick lenses. The abusive situation no longer exists, and he has moved out of his fearful approach to life and people. We are beginning to reduce his dependency and his prescription as we work together, but one can't help but wonder how much clearer his vision would be now if he'd had the help and encouragement that Olivia enjoys.

If Olivia had continued to wear those -4's all day, every day ... well, there isn't much doubt in my mind that her eyesight would be much worse as she entered adulthood, and her dependency on the lenses, much more pronounced. I shudder to think about it, having watched her quick improvement and knowing that she is now playing at the park on swings and playing ball games without lenses and without problems.

It is my passionate belief that the alternative of risk-free, Natural Vision practices should be in the hands of parents and educators so that more children can grow up knowing how to care for their precious eyes, for life. In learning and demonstrating this kind of care for their own eyes, parents become excellent role models, like Olivia's Mom and Dad have been, and continue to be, for her.

In the Dark

Children love to palm their eyes. When I first discovered this whole body of knowledge, I was working in a classroom, teaching Grade Three. I taught my students the why and the how of palming, and they gleefully participated in a palming period every day, after our silent reading was complete.

Once their eyes were covered and everybody was breathing deeply, I could actually feel the children's excitement about what would happen next. I would guide them to imagine that they were walking slowly down a staircase, becoming more and more relaxed, and then, when reaching the bottom where it was very dark, they would reach a magical kingdom.

In this place, I encouraged them to see lots of wonderful, imaginary things; some I suggested and some they invented themselves. The classroom was totally quiet and yet intense, while we would all palm and go to these wonderful imaginary places.

After a few minutes, I would have the children take their cupped hands away from their closed eyes, invite the light in, and then blink 20 - 30 times to stimulate their eye muscles and come back to "real" seeing.

Sometimes I would ask the children to then write stories or paint pictures of what they had just imagined and they would go to work very enthusiastically and intent on showing me what they had "seen" in their "mind's eyes".

Palming was always a good experience for them, and many of my students would tell me how they palmed their eyes before bed, or when they could feel that their eyes were tired. Children in our classroom were allowed and encouraged to palm their eyes when they felt any eye strain or fatigue. This kind of awareness is priceless, and how wonderful to be developing that kind of consciousness at age seven or eight!

Sometimes we would take the whole thing one step further. If there were disagreements/problems in our classroom, we would sometimes go to the dark space to find the answers. I remember that our class had created a beautiful "butterfly garden" outside as part of a science project and nature study. The girls were quite upset with the boys one day because the boys had been playing games in the garden that the girls felt were discouraging our hoped-for butterflies from visiting.

Everyone was ready for a big argument when the children came in from recess one day, so I suggested that instead of talking about the problem, we gather together and palm quietly and look inside for answers.

Everybody agreed on this idea and as we went into our dark palming space, I had the children imagine our garden with many butterflies of different colours all visiting the plants. As always, I could feel their excitement, visualizing these beautiful butterflies.

Then I asked them to ask the butterflies they were seeing in their mind's eyes why they had come there — what conditions made the garden attractive to them?

When we came out of palming, the hands flew up! Some butterflies wanted lots of water on the plants, some wanted quiet, some wanted music, some shade, some sunshine, some wanted activity and laughter, and on it went. We finally, happily decided that we could provide all of these situations in our garden and that could even include some boisterous play — just not all the time. So, on half the recesses, we left the garden alone and quiet, and the other ones, play was allowed.

This kind of experience teaches children so many things: that they can rely on their mind's imagination to help find answers to their questions, that settling down, being quiet, and breathing deeply helped to channel their anger towards a better resolution, and that by going inside for a minute, they might find something more constructive to contribute on the outside.

"Proof"

Recently it was reported that Canadian researchers did a study on kittens with amblyopia, or "lazy eye" as it is more commonly called. They simply placed the kittens in total darkness for ten days, and their eyes recovered.

The researchers at Dalhousie University made the statement that the darkness `had restored "brain plasticity": "Immersion in total darkness seems to reset the visual brain to enable remarkable recovery," they said. This type of research, recognizing the healing effects of darkness, is very hopeful for anyone looking for natural and risk-free steps to take towards eye health.

Although we don't want to be in darkness for ten days, why not just try darkness four times per day for a couple of minutes each time? My experience with many children has already shown me that that amount of darkness is helpful on many levels.

Physically, when palming is combined with good rest in a dark bedroom at night, a child's eyes are getting the rest required to meet the demands of busy days.

Nutrition for Demanding Eyes

For a growing child's eyes, nutrition plays a key role. Grandma was right; carrots are good for the eyes, especially for night vision, and so are many other commonly found foods, especially when the produce is as fresh as possible.

If you go through this list for your own benefit, or with your child, try to underline at least two foods that you commonly consume for each nutrient and then make a plan to try something new each week.

Making smoothies can be a wonderful way to blend flavours and disguise a bit of kale or spinach that might not be your first choice.

Here's the basic list of what eyes need for health and some common sources; (feel free to do some of your own research here; this is by no means the whole list!)

Vitamin A: carrots, butter, egg yolk, green, leafy vegetables

---

Vitamin B1:	beans, nuts, wheat germ, potatoes, broccoli
Vitamin B2:	yogurt, soybeans, spinach, almonds, eggs
Vitamin B12:	cheese, egg yolks, fish, meat, yeast
Vitamin C:	green leafy vegetables, potatoes, parsley, citrus fruit, strawberries
Vitamin E:	oils, nuts, seeds, wheat germ, green leafy vegetables
Calcium:	whole grains and cereals, milk products, green vegetables
Chromium	whole grain cereals, unsaturated fats, meats
Copper:	whole grain products, almonds, green leafy vegetables, seafood
Iron:	whole grain breads and cereals, fruits and vegetables
Magnesium:	nuts, whole grain foods, dry beans and peas, dark green vegetables, soy products

Manganese:	egg yolks, sunflower seeds, wheat germ, whole grain cereals and flour, dried peas and beans
Phosphorous:	whole grains, eggs, seeds, nuts, fish, meat
Selenium:	whole grain cereals, broccoli, onions, tomatoes and tuna
Potassium:	green leafy vegetables, whole grains, oranges, sunflower seeds, potatoes and bananas
Zinc:	beans, nuts, seeds, wheat germ, fish and meat

Patient Beware

All parents should take real care in the professional chosen to examine their child's eyes.

A university study conducted by Vanderbilt University School of Medicine and published in the *Journal of the American Association of Pediatric Ophthalmology and Strabismus,* provided some striking, if not shocking information.

The study reported the following for children under the care of an eye professional:

- Optometrists — prescribed glasses 35% of the time

- General Ophthalmologists — prescribed glasses 12% of the time

- **Pediatric Ophthalmologists — prescribed glasses only 2% of the time**

This study clearly shows the importance of choosing the right professional eye doctor. Plus, the study concluded that Optometrists and Ophthalmologists who usually treat adults "may not have as much expertise with children". (Well, yes.)

It appears that Pediatric Ophthalmologists are more cognizant of the fact that a growing child's eyes are very resilient and more than one examination might be in order, before making the decision to give the child prescription lenses.

It's a Good Idea to Have Fun!

Just a few decades previous to now, a typical child would get out of school where their eyes may have been busy with close work for many hours, and go home and play outdoors, swinging on swings, playing ball games, and other distance-seeing activities.

Nowadays, however, many children are playing with their electronic devices after school (even on the bus on the way home) for many more hours. This type of lifestyle places extreme stress on the eyes.

When I begin working with a child, some of the "homework" I assign gets the child outdoors and playing outdoor games. In every case I've seen, having to get out there and do these things results in the child going out and staying out for longer than I asked.

It's also great when a parent is part of the solution. Just playing catch with a ball or frisbee is of huge benefit to the eyes, because it gets them tracking visually, focusing at different distances, practicing hand/eye coordination, discerning detail, tracking contrasting colour, and more and all of this under the wonderful stimulation of the full-spectrum light.

And these activities can be done only for the fun and joy of the play; no competition required.

Healthy Vision in Our Classrooms

A passionate dream of mine is to introduce Natural Eye and Vision Care into the curriculums across the land. Back when I was teaching Health in Ontario, as part of my Health curriculum, I taught Care of the Teeth, Personal Hygiene, Canada's Food Rules and Nutrition, Our Digestive System, and probably a couple more units I have forgotten.

Aside from learning how our visual system functions and learning to name the parts of the eye, nothing is taught to young children about how to care for their eyes and prevent or correct situations of fatigue and stress. And yet, our very schools are where so much of the stress takes place. It seems to me that a discussion about preventative care naturally belongs in the educational system.

A very big part of a young child's education is, of course, teaching him/her how to read. Reading with fluency and understanding is one of life's important skills and also greatest pleasures. However, the child learning to read is new to this whole idea of staring at something very close for long periods of time.

The time it would take to teach children how to read in a relaxed posture and mind-set would be minimal, but could save those precious eyes from requiring the crutch of glasses. Pausing to palm, or look off into the distance to relax the eyes and stimulate them in a different way, is a habit

Joy Thompson

that we need to cultivate in our growing children and ourselves.

There is no question that looking off into the distance, or up at the sky, stimulates the imagination. I would ask my students to read a section of text, and then instruct them to palm their eyes or look out the window at something far away (their choice; either activity relaxes the eyes and therefore the body), and think about what they had just read. This extends the learning stimulated by what has been read ... and activates the child's ability to comprehend and imagine.

CHAPTER NINE

Complications

**"If the eye does not want to see, neither light
nor glasses will help"**
— German proverb

Our body creates millions of new cells every second. That means that you have generated many 100's of million new cells during the time it took you to read this sentence. This is a good bit of trivia to remember when we think of holistic healing ... we set the intention to heal, and then in cooperation with our minds, we provide our bodies with the opportunity to regenerate in a healthy way.

One of the many good reasons for keeping vision as sharp as possible all our lives is that eye disease doesn't seem to appear out of nowhere. It occurs usually in those who already have impaired vision and are doing nothing about it, probably because they simply don't know any healthy eye practices.

Think it over. Do you know anyone with excellent eyesight, who doesn't depend on lenses, who has an eye disease? William Bates tried to teach us that for eyes to stay healthy, they need to be exercising when they look, as they were designed to be. Relaxed eyes see well, can refocus quickly at many different distances, and make demands from a healthy body to fuel their work.

So, eyes that sit behind glasses all day, every day, and get a "free ride" are in danger of becoming lazy and unstimulated and yes, ill. Even someone who isn't using lenses is bound to have very tired, stressed eyes after decades of over-using them without any rest periods or targeted stimulation.

So, perhaps it's not so much aging that is the problem, but rather, years of neglect and overuse. And of course that brings us back to lack of education regarding what eyes need to stay healthy and function well, which is the reason for this book and others like it.

When we are ill, almost everyone agrees that we need rest in order to get better. My Mom was a nurse, and she would not tolerate anyone "trying to be a hero and making everyone else sick"... at the first sign of a cold, infection or 'flu, we were told to go to bed and rest because, she explained, rest is when the body can direct its energy towards getting healthy again.

Make sense? That idea has always made sense to me and I've been bewildered by those who have terrible colds or upset stomachs, or worse, and go off to work anyway, ignoring their ailing bodies.

If we accept the idea that rest enables healing, then we need to rest our eyes more when they are showing signs of stress. Stress can take many forms besides just blurriness — watering, bloodshot, aching, a feeling of scratchiness, like sand in the eye, styes, iritis, conjunctivitis, and on it goes.

When these more minor (although not minor to the sufferer) irritations come along, it might be a good idea to take an inventory of the places in your life that are irritating you. I say this because everyone I've met who suffers from styes or "itis-es" is usually also irritated, and sometimes chronically. Our eyes are simply mirrors of our feelings in many cases — and if we can solve the problem emotionally, it really helps to soothe us physically as well. It's worth pondering.

Joy Thompson

I've been called on dozens of occasions by people who have any of the above conditions, and every time I tell people how to palm and rest their eyes, and suggest they get lots of rest/sleep in a darkened room. Sometimes these conditions require medication from the doctor, of course, but it only stands to reason that rest will help the medicine work as well.

One other helpful hint for stressed eyes is to place a clean, cold and wet, folded washcloth over closed eyes and lie down for awhile. The coolness is very refreshing, and I do that once a day for my own eyes, "palming" without using my hands.

Palming before and after any surgical procedure is of course a good idea, as well as palming before visiting the Optometrist for an examination. In all these situations, we want our eyes as relaxed as possible.

Cataracts

A cataract means that the crystalline lens of the eye, through which we look, is becoming cloudy. The most common symptom is of course, blurry, clouded vision.

Over 300,000 Canadians suffer from cataracts, which can eventually result in blindness. Cataract surgery has become the most common surgery performed on those over 65 years of age.

Margaret's Story

Margaret was 77 when she contacted me — on the day she cancelled her cataract surgery. She said that she believed whole-heartedly in self-healing and she was sure she could work towards eliminating her cataracts without surgery.

She said that she had several pairs of glasses for different seeing situations — a pair she used for distance, a pair for computer work, another pair for reading music as she played the piano, and also a pair of bifocals that she didn't like much. She was ready to "clear all this up".

Margaret was ready to get started, but I was a little hesitant; I had never begun with someone on the day they were scheduled for surgery and I was concerned that if surgery was warranted, the cataracts must be pretty serious. Margaret insisted that they weren't bothering her and she wanted to explore self-healing of her eyes before she did something as radical as having her lenses replaced.

So, the next week, with some trepidation on my part, we began with an assessment. Margaret told me that her Ophthalmologist's office had called her twice, trying to reschedule the surgery, and again, I wondered how serious this was.

My fears were soon allayed. Margaret could read down three lines on my eye chart with no problem at all. I "tested" her with several other questions, but her answers were not at all typical of someone with cataracts. It seemed that there was no serious visual loss as she was managing just fine, but was tired of using glasses.

What Margaret was experiencing was some long-standing myopia, some presbyopia, and some astigmatism in her left eye.

We got to work. Margaret was not only coopera-tive; on most days, she was way ahead of me. She did an enormous amount of reading on the subject of Natural Vision Improvement, and she completed all the practices I gave her as well as others she was learning about from her reading.

Margaret was already supplementing with Bilberry*, believed to be a cataract deterrent, and her diet was really excellent. She added some other supplements as well as time went by, did her exer-cises and was obviously enjoying the whole process. She didn't seem to doubt for a second that she had made the right decision to delay surgery.

We reduced the strength of the glasses Margaret was using at all distances. Margaret doesn't drive a car, so there was no issue around driving safety. She used pinhole glasses daily for reading instead of her prescription lenses. Also, Margaret went for some period each day without any glasses, and she enjoyed the "impressionistic painting" that was her home without lenses.

Exactly fourteen months later, Margaret visited an Optometrist I recommended — someone I knew would examine her carefully without rushing the appointment, and would be willing to prescribe lenses of a strength that would be therapeutic for her.

After a very thorough examination, the Optometrist declared that there was only a "bit of cataract" in one of her eyes, "but nothing to worry about, and certainly not requiring surgery"! Woo-hoo! Margaret's vision had improved at every distance, and she was given a prescription for the lenses that she is using sometimes now, with no astigmatism correction.

There are two possibilities here; either she was misdiagnosed with cataracts in the first place, or she had them before and now they were almost completely gone. We'll never know for sure, but what is sure, is that this clever lady avoided unnecessary surgery.

Now, at 79, Margaret's eyes are better than ever! Please pause for a moment here, especially if you are someone who laments that we deteriorate as we age. What Margaret accomplished defies this idea completely and she is made out of the same stuff as the rest of us.

I'm not at all suggesting that others scheduled for cataract surgery should cancel. I am definitely saying that there are two important points of view with any surgery; the viewpoint of the surgeon, and that of the patient.

At the end of the day of surgery, it is the patient who has been altered, and therefore the patient who must make all the final, and hopefully, fully informed, decisions — no one else.

* (One study of 50 patients showed that bilberry extracts plus vitamin-E stopped progression of cataract formation in 97 percent of patients with age related cataracts. Bilberry , some evidence suggests, also helps to improve night vision. The usual dose is 40 to 80 mgs of bilberry per day. I take 40 mg. per day.)

Blindness

As it happens, one of my very first clients had an extremely rare degenerative eye disease. He had always been slightly myopic, but now had been declared legally blind, because the "black holes" in his field of vision were obscuring his seeing to an enormous extent. He could discern well enough to work and use public transit, but could no longer drive.

He was completely disenchanted with the medical establishment in his country and not ready to accept the fact that he would soon be completely blind and there was absolutely nothing that could be done.

We worked together over the course of one year, during which time he reported that his visual field had increased and he was more confident in discerning light and shadow. His myopia decreased measurably and he was again able to read the train schedules at the station, and was delighted with this improvement. He felt better and more optimistic and that was significant, as his diagnosis of impending blindness had put him into a tailspin that bordered on depression a lot of the time.

Now he was smiling and speaking positively, and enjoying the vision practices even for their own sake and the sense of strong relief he felt at participating in a program designed to stimulate his eyesight.

That was many years ago now, but it was wonderful to be a part of his success and particularly to know that all he was doing was risk-free and pro-active.

This "nothing can be done" diagnosis dismays me to no end. As I keep repeating, palming can be done, stimulating with gentle sunlight can be done, reviewing one's diet and improving it can be done, visualizations can be done, perhaps some supplements can be used that appear helpful — just for starts.

What happens here, through the doing, is that hope arrives. Hope is not to be dismissed as silly or inconsequential! Someone's hope has been the beginning of any positive change anyone can name, and no one can predict just how far hope can take us! Let's enlist it and use it, for heaven's sake.

Glaucoma

Glaucoma is a sneaky eye disease that seems to creep up. It is caused by a pressure build up in the vitreous fluid of the eyes.

It's almost as though the eyes are a pressure-cooker, building and building pressure, and the danger of glaucoma unchecked is permanent vision loss. In the two cases I've worked with, the doctors were keeping close tabs on their patients, checking pressures regularly. At a certain high point, surgery might have been necessary to reduce the intra-ocular pressures.

So in taking the natural approach to try to help in both cases, my clients began to palm their eyes for fairly long periods (20 minutes or more) several times each day, and also, once a day, would lie down with a cold cloth placed over their closed eyes. Visualizing serene vistas while breathing deeply was also a part of the palming regimen.

Then, we gradually added some very gentle eye movement to stimulate without stressing the eyes.

I suggested they eliminate or greatly reduce their caffeine and alcohol intake, and get very light but enjoyable exercise daily. They also each kept a journal, writing down any areas in their lives where they felt "pressured" and took whatever steps they could to reduce this. We talked about all of this and any other concerns at length on a weekly basis.

In the first case, the man reduced his pressures from 25 in the right and 22 in the left (high), to 15 and 14 in each eye, (normal) respectively, over a six month period.

I cannot guarantee that the work we did together was the cause of this, but my client certainly believed it was. He still has regular checkups and his pressures today, 12 years later, remain in the normal, safe range.

This past year, I used roughly the same program with a woman whose pressure was over 30 in one eye — very high, and concerning for her and her doctor. She wanted to participate in her own healing, and followed the regimen daily for four months, until her next checkup. She also used some natural eye drops she had found that seemed to help and from our understanding, certainly couldn't hurt.

After the four months, she found that her eye pressures were reduced to the low 20's, much to everyone's relief, and she still continues her Natural Vision practices and works to keep stress to a minimum in her life.

Retinitis Pigmentosa

This disorder is characterized by the progressive loss of retinal cells and may eventually lead to blindness. I have not been contacted by anyone with retinitis pigmentosa … that was a possibility in Daniel's diagnosis, but the conclusion was never a firm one.

Grace's Story

I read Grace Halloran's book, "Amazing Grace" years ago, when I was reading and digesting everything I could about Natural Vision Improvement. The story within those pages was so fascinating, I feel it merits mentioning here.

Grace Halloran was diagnosed with Retinitis Pigmentosa and Macular Degeneration in the early 1970's. She was 23. She was also told that her infant son would go blind early in life as well, as he appeared to have inherited the same condition.

Grace began a life-long search for help in eye conditions that have traditionally been labeled untreatable and incurable. To that end, she earned her PhD from Columbia Pacific University in Holistic Health Science.

Grace's program used the technology of microcurrent stimulation for the treatment of eye disease at her education centre in California, and she recorded many successes there. Her own vision improved, and by the latest reports, her son's vision did not deteriorate.

Grace's book, *"Amazing Grace — Autobiography of a Survivor"*, was selected by the Easter Seal Society and the American Library Association as one of the best inspirational books on the market in 2001. It certainly inspired me.

Grace Halloran taught her Integrated Visual Healing Program to hundreds of individuals all over the world.

Sadly, in 1986, Grace was exposed to extensive radiation from the Chernobyl disaster. She never completely recovered, and died in 2005.

Aging Eyes

I see no reason whatsoever why we cannot have very healthy eyes for our entire lifetimes, and indeed, many people do. Decades of neglect and overuse and strain can account for problems, but if we know what we are doing and take good care of our eyes, we make it easy for them to perform well. Besides just attending to the physical factors, we need to take a look at what we are habitually thinking as well.

Our eyes see better when we are excited and full of anticipation. An article in Scientific American magazine in August, 2013, cites a study that "proves" this idea with some interesting data. Here's the article, verbatim:

Can our thoughts improve our vision? We tend to believe that an essentially mechanical process determines how well we see. Recent research by Ellen Langer and colleagues suggests otherwise.

It is a common belief that fighter pilots have very good vision. The researchers put people in the mindset of an Air Force pilot by bringing them into a flight simulator. The simulator consisted of an actual cockpit including flight instruments. The cockpit was mounted on hydraulic lifts that mimic aircraft movement and performance. People were given green army fatigues; they sat in the pilot's seat, and performed simple flight maneuvers. They took a vision test while "flying" the simulator. A control group took the same vision test in the cockpit while the simulator was inactive. People's vision improved only if they were in the working simulator.

To rule out the possible effect of motivation, the researchers brought another group of people into the cockpit and asked them to read a brief essay on motivation. After people finished reading, they were strongly urged to be as motivated as possible and try hard to perform well in the vision test. The test was conducted

Joy Thompson

while the simulator was inactive. They did not show a significant improvement.

So part of what can be learned from this study is that when the test subjects had something really meaningful and exciting to do, they were seeing well or actually, better than normal. This shows us what many of us already know, intuitively; we must stay fully engaged in life to keep enjoying it as we get older, and find activities that excite us.

Too often, people limit themselves because of their age, saying they can't start something new because of it. But many others are blowing the limits off that kind of thinking every day, and to fully discuss this subject would require another book ... but let's just agree that to age well, we must keep our minds sharp, keep ourselves happy and keep engaged in life. We need to do this for many reasons, not the least of which being that this kind of thinking will actually help to keep eyesight clear.

In the western world, we have come to value youth almost to ridiculous proportions. Elders in society should be enjoyed and respected for their wisdom and wit, rather than being ignored or forgotten.

However, I will add that in becoming elders, we have our own responsibility to stay worthy of respect. We need to respect ourselves first and then cultivate the expectation that we will age with panache and grace and health!

Expectations affect eyesight, and Ellen Langer went on to prove that with a further study:

In an eye exam, we are used to experiencing problems at the bottom third of the eye chart, where letters start to get small. In another experiment, Ellen Langer and colleagues showed people a shifted chart. At the top, it included letters equivalent to the medium-size letters on the normal eye chart and the chart progressed to letters of very small size at the bottom. Because people were expecting to read the top two thirds of the shifted chart as well, they were able to read much smaller letters.

This is amazing data, and is proof that our expectations are enormous factors in the results we achieve (or don't achieve).

If people expect their vision to remain keen or to improve, it will, at least to some extent. And it also follows that, if we believe that our vision will deteriorate and we are powerless to make any changes, that's very likely to come true for us as well.

Which would you prefer to be right about?

Just imagine a culture where we are told repeatedly that as we age we become more and more like fine wine; the older the vintage, the better! Imagine magazine and movie images of older people with naturally lined faces, appreciated because of their obvious experience and age.

Imagine being told by professionals that physical ailments that we might be experiencing could improve as we make changes that pave the way for natural health.

As a result, people might stop obsessing about looking younger and stop spending so much time and billions of dollars on that ridiculous pursuit. And what's more wonderful — they could begin to value their experience and older appearance, and the wisdom of their developing consciousness.

We could actually become proud of ourselves and the way we look and feel as we move through life at any stage. This doesn't mean that there aren't challenges and difficulties along the way; just that we are confident that we will move through them and expand and grow as a result.

We need to consider what a privilege it is to live to grow older, period.

I completely believe that our eyes can stay healthy as we get older, and in the past 18 years, that's been my own experience, and I've seen improvement and stabilization now with many hundreds of others. I've also watched clients develop more confidence, more understanding and more self-assurance as they consider an improvement in their seeing and therefore, their world-view, literally and figuratively.

Native elders, shamanic teachers, yogis, and other leaders have come and gone and given us fantastic examples of not just aging gracefully, but with panache and class — giving back so much before leaving us.

So please, let's stop making fun of ourselves! You know, all the familiar comments that because we're older we don't look as good, can't see, hear, think, remember etc. etc. What poor jokes these are! Living longer doesn't have to equal any of these things so perhaps we should stop talking that way and poking fun at others and ourselves.

As cited above, what we believe tends to be what comes true for us.

Let's replace our fears with acceptance, excitement, and celebration and learn to love ourselves and others at every stage. We can continually look for possibilities and find hope and excitement waiting there.

We can each make that choice today.

CHAPTER TEN

Lighting Up

"We can easily forgive a child who is afraid of the dark; the real tragedy of life, is when we are afraid of the Light."
— Plato

As we improve our vision naturally, we can count on more dialog between our eyes and our bodies, and this has an enormous positive side to it, as the pleasure and satisfaction that we feel in our bodies when happy and contented, courses through us and shines from our eyes. We can revel in that feeling of satisfaction and pleasure.

Dr. Alexander Lowen, one of my favourite authors, and a pioneer in studying the field of Bionergetics, wrote this in his wonderful book, *The Spirituality of the Body*:

> "It is the eyes that inevitably reveal the difference between a genuine smile and a mask. A genuine smile is the result of a wave of excitation that flows upward, brightening the face and lighting up the eyes, just as a house lights up when someone is home."

He goes on to say:

> "When I was a medical student studying Ophthalmology, I opened my textbook to find the statement, "The eyes are the mirrors of the soul". I was excited by the prospect of learning more about this aspect of the eyes, but the words "mirror" and "soul" were never mentioned again. Science is interested only in the mechanical functioning of the organs, not in their inherent spirituality. If something cannot be measured, it cannot be dealt with scientifically. We have no way to measure soulfulness objectively, or love or hate. Yet, we have all been regarded by loving eyes, hateful eyes, soulful eyes. We know beyond the shadow of a doubt that all these intangible (and immeasurable) qualities exist."

Remembering that the brain and eye are basically one and the same, since retinal tissue is brain tissue, it makes perfect sense that what enters through our eyes touches every part of us.

The Museum of Vision says:

"One layer of the retina is brain tissue which begins coding visual information even before messages are sent via the optic nerve to the brain."

So, just as what we are thinking affects the way we see, what we are seeing affects our thoughts and our entire body, since all is completely connected through the web of our nervous system.

If we see a child run in front of a bus, our nervous and circulatory systems react right away and we immediately run to pull the child to safety. In seeing someone we love after a long separation, we are compelled to move with great energy as well, only this time, motivated by joy rather than fear — but the energy is the same and our eyes compel it.

Most of us have had the joyful experience of watching a baby take his/her first steps. The child looks at us as we extend our arms, saying, "C'mon, sweetie, come here" and the child looks intensely at us as he/she takes those first awkward steps forward. There is real tension in the child's eyes; those eyes are saying, "Stay right there and look at me and while we keep this strong eye contact, I feel safe in moving forward." If something disturbs this connection, even for a second, the child will plop right back on the floor. He is **holding on** with his eyes, using the connection to move himself forward and stay upright.

That's a healthy, safe way to use your eyes and to learn to walk when you are 12 months old, and once he's mastered the skill, his eyes will relax once again.

However, if we are looking at everything with that kind of underlying fear, and all that tension, we can't create safety in the long term, and eventually our eyes will tire out from over-focusing all the time. Many people look at life in this tense, controlling way, and the letting go can be frightening in the beginning, but is more than worthwhile.

The Meridian System

The ancient art and science of the Energy Meridian system teaches that the energy, or chi, in our body moves along through pathways. Collectively these pathways form the matrix within which our physical body functions.

The Meridians have been acknowledged for thousands of years, and are verified and used today in the practices of qigong, acupuncture, acupressure, tai chi, and the newer, very popular practice of EFT.

Five major energy meridians complete in the eyes and are affected by them ... The liver, heart, gall bladder, bladder and stomach meridians.

Liver is the organ of passion in both positive (love, creativity and excitement) and negative (anger) forms. Most of us remember the power of the "evil eye" from an angry parent or teacher that zapped us, even decades ago. Liver energy also translates to passion and love for someone or something, and we all know how these feelings sparkle in the eyes of the passionate ones.

The bladder meridian has been associated with fear on the negative side, and its positive opposite, determined resolution. A commonly used example of this: a mother finds her child pinned under a car and her first feeling is extreme terror, followed quickly by a strong resolution that she will save her child. Through this feeling of determination she commands enough energy and strength into her limbs and muscles to actually lift the car off her child.

As mentioned before, fear is often locked into our eyes in the form of tension, and this tension can be coaxed away through physical movement, relaxation techniques, and reassurance in different forms. Once we have processed any fears that might be keeping us frozen in the fear response, we can transform the energy of fear into a forward-moving energy of "resolution".

Sometimes we need help to get out of "fear" mode; especially if we were frozen in a fearful place as children, and now need to "thaw out" in order to move forward. Many people don't feel their fears and so are painfully unaware of how fear is directing their lives.

In working with softening and relaxing the eyes, a fear will occasionally present itself, as in the case of my daughter and her vague fears about seeing in the distance. Often, all that is needed is a little dialog and reassurance that there is no longer any threat "out there". If someone is willing to accept that and has resolved to see with courage, they are well on their way to clearing the old, outdated and no-longer-required blur.

The stomach meridian is associated with irritation/ revulsion on the negative side and contentment/ satisfaction on the positive. Most of us can recall a time when we saw something that made our "stomach turn" in revulsion; the link between the eyes and the stomach cannot be denied, and yet, as we age, many of us develop the ability to look at horrific scenes — on the news or in violent movies or TV shows — without the slightest body reaction. The eyes have detached from the body in such cases, and not necessarily in a positive way.

Who is more emotionally healthy? Someone who turns off their television in response to a feeling of revulsion in their stomach when seeing a violent scene, or the person who looks at such horror and feels nothing at all?

When we see something that is highly pleasing to us, a feeling of contentment and pleasure settles in our bellies, and we can revel in that lovely sensation that all is well with the world.

One branch of the heart meridian runs through the throat and up into the eyes. How often do we have the experience of feeling highly touched emotionally, feeling a lump in our throat and tears welling up in our eyes all at the same time? This is the experience of seeing with our hearts.

A constricted throat and jaw area can limit energy moving back and forth from the heart and eyes, and so I encourage clients to open their throats through chanting or singing as well as massage, in order to keep that channel as clear as possible. Cultivating the habit of talking about feelings or "talking through" problems can help to keep the throat open and the energy moving.

I like to imagine that as positive energy moves freely along the meridians, it is analogous to tiny lights enlivening the body and brightening the eyes ...

I once had a client who worked diligently on her vision exercises without much change in her eyesight until one day, a sad memory from her childhood surfaced. She told me all about the heartbreak of so many years ago, and how sad and abandoned she'd felt. In talking about this, she began to sob almost uncontrollably, and that crying kept surfacing and retreating for a couple of days, until finally, she seemed to have "unloaded" all the sadness associated with the memories.

The next time we measured her vision, we confirmed what she already knew; that she was seeing much better and more clearly than in many years, having unloaded so much old tension that had been locked into her face and eyes. I noticed that her eyes appeared to be a clearer blue than ever before, and there was a liveliness to her eyes and body that was lovely to witness. She also appeared much younger than when we had begun our work together.

Part of the Whole

If we look at eyes and vision in a holistic way, we cannot see them as orbs that sit in our face and are not connected to the rest of us. And yet, it seems as though medical science does treat eyes as though treating and changing their configuration has no affect on our whole selves. But subjective evidence that every one of us has felt on more than one occasion tells us another story.

It is my absolute belief that eyes can show us the level of energy flowing easily within a person. A happy baby's eyes shine so gloriously that we gather 'round in big crowds just to get a glimpse of them. Compare that child's eyes with those of a severely depressed person sitting alone in the hospital. The contrast is huge.

There is just no question that we see more clearly when we are happy, when we are looking forward to something, when we are physically fit, when we are well nourished, and when we are feeling love.

Our eyes see and reveal it all.

CHAPTER ELEVEN

Our Bodies and Our Eyes

"I think that the ideal space must contain elements of magic, serenity, sorcery and mystery."
— Luis Barragan

Based on my knowledge of vision improvement, yoga, bioenergetics and meditation practices, I created a workshop, which is outlined right here in this chapter. It includes many easy movements, stretches and postures that, when practiced regularly for just a few minutes each day, support health and healing of the eyes, as well as creating better body posture and a stronger body/mind connection.

It's all connected ... as Bates told us: "It is not possible to have a completely healthy body with eyes that are ill, and vice-versa." Again, this is a natural process so it takes time, but within about three days of doing the practices below, you'll probably feel better, and that's the sign that you are doing something right!

To work really well, our bodies need strong and flexible muscles, a good digestive system, a strong cardiovascular system, an alert brain, and so much more, as well as an optimally functioning pair of eyes communicating, through its very close connection along the optic nerve, to our brain.

First, we want to develop the ability to relax deeply through breathing practices and meditative states. Those practices prepare the body for strengthening and increased flexibility.

If you can, claim a quiet area somewhere in your home to do this practice daily. There's more "magic" in a space that you have created with deliberate intent; perhaps a lit candle, flowers, some incense or burning oils, a special mat or blanket, soft music or simply quiet. It's your space — make it special so that your time there feels intentional and personal.

* * * * *

Please read first:

Read through all the instructions first with each description. Read one line and just close your eyes and think about yourself doing what has been described. Then go on, line by line, visualizing before you do anything. Visualizing will help enormously in your understanding of each movement or practice and will help to make each exercise your own.

Also please note:

** People with glaucoma, detached retina, high blood pressure, or people who often suffer from dizziness should NOT do any of the **inverted positions, because such positions can be too stimulating. Anything here that is not inverted, however, should be safe.

If you're unsure, talk to your health caregiver.

* * * * *

Shoulder openers:

These three movements can be done as you begin the regimen below, or just for their own sake. I do these three exercises when I take breaks from working at the computer, because desk work tends to restrict the upper body especially.

These practices help keep us aware, relaxed and alive.

Close your eyes, if you wish, while doing the upper body relaxers ...

1. Sitting on a chair, bring your shoulders up as high as possible, towards your ears. Hold for a minute and feel the whole area becoming very tense. Take a deep breath in, and then exhale loudly as you let your shoulders drop and relax. Repeat a few times.

** (INVERSION)

2. Push your chair away from your desk and place your feet flat on the floor, shoulder-width apart. Bend forward and let your head hang down loosely. Breathe deeply and slowly. Feel your back and neck lengthen as you breathe.

3. Sitting up, reach out in front of you, and then bend your arms and cross them over each other. Place your right hand on your left shoulder and your left hand on your right shoulder, giving yourself a "hug". Breathe fully and feel your upper back open.

Alternate Nostril Breathing

Sit in a comfortable position and take in a few deep breaths. Now, with one finger, close your right nostril and take three full, deep breaths through your left nostril. Then, close your left nostril and take three breaths through your right. Complete with three long, slow breaths through both nostrils.

Swaying

Swaying is described fully in Chapter Six. When I teach a yoga class, I always begin with swaying, to loosen the back, shoulders and to quiet the mind and relax vision in preparation for the yoga postures. You could play some background music to help relax you while swaying.

Lower Back Stretch

Lie down on your back and get into a deep breathing rhythm. Imagine and feel all of your back muscles softening as you accept the support of the floor underneath you. Now bend your legs and bring your knees up to your chest, grasping your legs behind the knees with your hands. Feel that great stretch in your lower back. Rock side to side, thereby giving your lower back a gentle massage as it stretches and you release and relax.

** (INVERSION) **Forward Bend**

Standing with legs about six inches apart, centre the weight of your body on the balls of your feet. Inhale deeply as you stretch both arms straight up over your head. Imagine your entire body extending upward. Exhale, stretching downward towards the floor. Grab hold of the back of your legs and feel the connection of your feet resting on the floor. Breathe and let your head hang down loosely, getting the sense of your neck lengthening, and back muscles benefitting with this stretch. Stay in forward bend for about one minute.

** (INVERSION) **Downward Dog**

While still in forward bend position, place your hands flat on the floor, bending your knees if necessary. Move your feet well back, one at a time until your body is in an "inverted V" position. Let your head hang loosely. Feel the support of your hands and feet. Breathe deeply and stay in this position for a minute or two. (the name "downward dog" is an apt one — my dog does this stretch every morning!)

Cobra

Lie on your stomach, face down on your mat with eyes closed. Breathe deeply and bring your focus to your body. Now bring your arms forward as you raise your upper back. With your entire forearms and both elbows placed underneath your chest to support you, look straight ahead while bringing your attention to the space between your two eyes. Breathe deeply and hold this posture and attention for a minute or two.

Simple Twist

Sit on the floor with your legs straight out in front of you. Bend your right knee, placing your right foot flat on the floor on the outside of your left knee. Now, turn your upper body to the right, placing your hands comfortably on the floor for support. Look far to the right, feeling the twist in your back and neck as you look far to the right. Reverse and repeat, looking to the left side.

** (INVERSION) Triangle

(It might be helpful to begin by standing with a wall behind you for support.)

Stand up and plant your feet hip-width apart. Step forward with your right foot and reach your right arm down towards your foot. Your left arm is stretched up towards the sky. Look up at your left hand and breathe deeply and focus.

Repeat this sequence on the other side.

Eye Muscle Stretch

Sit or stand comfortably. Looking straight ahead, look up, (just by moving your eyes, not your head) as high as you can, down low, and then looking to each side. Feel your eye muscles get a good stretch. Palm for a minute to rest your eyes after this stretching practice.

Candle gazing

Sit comfortably, and place a lit candle at arm's length away from you at eye level. Gaze at the flame for about three minutes. If your eyes tire, just close them for a few seconds and you will still see the image of the flame with your eyes closed. I like to have soft music playing while I practice this focused concentration. It's okay to blink lots to keep your eyes lubricated while focusing.

Eye Lift

To improve or prevent 'heavy lidded-ness' as I've named it ... where the skin above the eye begins to droop down and weighs on the eyelids, giving us a "sleepy look", here's a simple exercise to do daily that will keep your eyebrows up high:

Lay the sides of your two pointer fingers, bent slightly to follow the length of your eyebrow arch, against your eyebrows, with tips of the fingers pointing towards each other. Press firmly against the eyebrows to keep them in place. Now blink and scrunch your eyes a bit. Hold the blink as you count 1, 2, 3, 4, 5 and then open your eyes wide. Repeat five times but hold to the count of ten on the last long blink.

Eye Massage

The technique for eye massage is described fully in Chapter Six. After all that you have just completed, energy is moving in your body and your eyes. Eye massage helps to relax and stimulate those tiny muscles supporting your eyes and vision and is a good final practice before palming.

Palming

To finish, palm and visualize something that makes you feel very happy and focus inward, on the happy feeling ... just breathing joy in and out. If visualizing makes you want to smile, so much the better. Smiling tells our brain, body, and being that all is well.

And truly, it is! You are moving along on the path of wellness!

Sometimes it's very nice to complete with a hot epsom salt bath if you can. The salt helps to draw out tensions as you bathe. It's also lovely to also add some aromatic oils to the bath, and to really spoil yourself, brew your favourite tea or make a smoothie to sip, light some candles and play some soft music while you soak.

Allow your body and eyes to take a "time out" as you relax and let go. You'll be glad that you gave this to yourself.

Practices like this don't take you away from more important work. They enhance your ability to come back to your activities renewed and refreshed, so that you can be the productive, creative and healthy soul that you were meant to be.

CHAPTER TWELVE

Profound Sight

"*All truth passes through three stages. First, it is ridiculed. Second, it is violently opposed. Third, it is accepted as being self-evident.*"
— Arthur Schopenhauer

I've spent my life enthusiastically learning things and then excitedly organizing what I've learned into a format that I can then teach to others. As I've stated before, no material I've come across in my lifetime has excited me more than the ideas and the possibilities that are inherent in the study of Natural Vision Improvement.

What holds me, and keeps me working and talking and studying, though, are the stories and the accomplishments of people I've worked with over the years. It's not just about being disciplined and committed, but about the exciting and courageous events that often accompany the improvement.

So rather than talk about the stories, I'll let them speak for themselves. I have not embellished anything here, because I believe the truth is dramatic enough in these cases.

The Story of Martha

Martha was a lovely, gentle woman who came to me when she was off work on disability benefits. She had been in a very high-stress job, and had finally collapsed and been diagnosed with Chronic Fatigue Syndrome. Doctor's orders were for her to be off work for at least six months, at which time he would re-evaluate the situation. Martha of course had very little energy, but was concerned about her failing vision and wanted to use some of her time off work to correct that, if possible.

Martha's right eye could see clearly but showed definite signs of fatigue. Her left eye was much weaker and overall, both eyes were seeing more and more blur at almost all distances. In her words, "I'm always looking through fog".

I initially gave Martha a lot of relaxation practices that would benefit her body as well as her eyes, because although she was very tired and in bed long hours; 12 - 14 hours each day, she was never refreshed by resting or sleeping.

Once Martha began to feel the benefits of focused relaxation, we started with exercises meant to stimulate her eyes to work together more cooperatively, and her visual acuity began to improve.

Once we had made some gains as far as Martha's clarity improving, I suggested that she spend 90 minutes or so each day with a patch over her right eye, in safe situations. Wearing a patch as part of a Vision Improvement program can help to rest the tired eye, and stimulate the weaker seeing eye to work a bit harder.

Martha's response to this suggestion made a lot of difference towards her reclaiming good vision. She was very committed to the idea, and every single day, she drove to her favourite forest trail, put the patch on her right eye, and then walked for the full 90 minutes, looking only with her left eye. She loved these walks ... saying the world "looked like a soft water-colour painting" that way.

Martha, it turned out, was a talented water-colour artist, and one day she gave me one of her beautiful paintings as a gift. I knew that she dreaded the thought of going back to her stressful job so I suggested that maybe she could try selling some of her paintings. Martha was absolutely sure that she could not make money from her art, telling me about all the talented artists she knew who were struggling. She said she also thought that making money from her work might take the enjoyment out of it.

After about six weeks of wearing a patch over her right eye every single day, followed by palming and blinking (to re-integrate the eyes and stimulate them), Martha came home from her walk and made some tea, as was her habit. She curled up in front of her fireplace.

As she told me later: "Suddenly, I could 'see' in my mind's eye, directly in front of me, a whole series of paintings of the forest. I knew with my whole heart that I would paint them ... I would do a series called 'Forest Moods' and paint the forest after the rain, in bright sunlight, in different seasons, and all the scenes that I knew so well from my walks. I could 'see' a gallery filled with my paintings and people coming to my showing."

She went on, enthused: "I wanted to finish my tea, but couldn't! I was so excited that I went downstairs to my little studio and got started right away! And I can't stop painting, suddenly; only long enough for meals and for my walks each day, but really, it's like these paintings are almost painting themselves and I'm just holding the brush! I was standing in my studio last week, working on a canvas and I realized that I was feeling something I hadn't felt in years. It was joy. I've been feeling really, truly happy," she beamed.

About three months later, Martha had completed twelve paintings and easily found a gallery to show her work. She sold four paintings at the showing, and then was able to sell some that were used as part of a display in a local restaurant.

Martha was feeling stronger all the time, and had renewed vigour thanks to adding some passion and purpose to her life. She was able to stop patching as both of her eyes improved and her seeing was more balanced overall, and certainly clearer.

Martha returned to her job after six months, but only working half-time hours, and she's painting (and selling paintings) with her free time, and her life appears to have found a much happier and healthier balance as well.

* * *

It is fairly accepted that the left eye stimulates the right brain (generally, our more artistic side) and the right eye stimulates the left brain (generally more mathematical), so it makes some sense that getting the eyes working naturally (without lenses) as well as possible, and as much as possible, helps to stimulate the whole brain.

My theory is that after a few weeks of stimulating some dormant parts of her brain through patching, Martha was able to have more of her own intelligence involved in her imagination and in her decision-making; intelligence that she hadn't been able to access through use of her weakened eyes and body. This expansion is what led to the breakthrough she experienced in envisioning her gallery showing, and subsequently marshaling enough physical energy to make it happen in reality.

* * *

The Story of Alex

Alex was 33 years old when I met him. He came to me very determined to "do something about" his rapidly increasing myopia. He was quite nearsighted and also had astigmatism in both eyes. He explained that he would have preferred to have laser surgery and just "get it done", but he was terrified of any kind of medical procedure and so there he was, staring at me with steel-grey eyes that demanded that I help him to see more clearly. Now.

Alex was a very intense person, not given to smiles or making little silly jokes (as I am), or to laughing at mine, but I liked him immediately, and I could sense a strong spirit looking directly at me.

So, we got to work. The first lesson was in palming and relaxing Alex's eyes. I took him through a very long, relaxing palming session, asking him to visualize a place that made him feel happy and contented. He chose his birthplace in Greece for this and all other visualizations, and I watched his face and body relax and soften noticeably while he was visualizing.

Alex and his parents had left Greece when he was only a boy - 9 years of age, but the impact on his life, I learned, had been enormous. His parents had presented a holiday to him, so he climbed aboard the Air Canada plane excited about the first vacation of his life.

But mid-way on the flight, somewhere over the Atlantic Ocean, his parents told him the truth; they would not be returning home, but instead had made extensive plans to make their new home in Canada, without his knowledge. Alex's emotions went from excitement to disbelief and then to absolute horror in a very short time, realizing that he would not be returning to his extended family (including his much-loved grandparents), his friends, everything he knew, and that he was about to land in a country he knew nothing about. He felt terrified and powerless, and that feeling stayed with him for decades.

That first year in Canada was horrible for Alex, and by age 10 he needed to wear glasses all the time in order to function at school. As I could only imagine, life had been very difficult for this young and very reluctant immigrant boy, trying to fit into Canadian society. Alex never adjusted to the much cooler Canadian climate and yearned for the tropical heat of his home country.

Alex was very bright in school, and as his grades improved with his English, his myopia increased. Now, at age 33, he was determined to stop the deterioration of his vision. He loved the palming sessions, and would always tell me afterwards how warm and relaxed he felt. "This is such a great feeling," he said, and I explained that it was the feeling of return to clarity. "First, it's just an occasional feeling, but later, it becomes your reality," I said. Alex was encouraged.

I saw Alex regularly for eight months, and at the beginning, as his vision slowly began to improve, he told me about feelings of anger that kept surfacing ... anger at his parents for deceiving him, anger at not being allowed to express his feelings openly, and very strong anger about living in Canada when he definitely wanted to be back in Greece. I suggested to him that he could go anytime — he was a grown man with skills he could use in his home country — he no longer was bound to staying. Alex was quick to give me a list of reasons why he couldn't go back; his girlfriend didn't want to leave Canada, he would have to start again with his career, his parents were aging and they were now Canadian citizens, etc. etc. so I didn't persist, but Alex continued to be angry, generally. As he expressed to me one day, "I'm just mad at everybody and everything some days, and I feel like I'm going to blow!"

Alex continued to work with his vision and to make real progress. Soon he was wearing a prescription that was half what we began with, and for a good part of each day he went without glasses at all. I encouraged him to do sunning practices to stimulate his eyes with light and he continued to love to palm, and would for long periods, "seeing" in his mind's eye his homeland in the blazing sun. He loved the hot sun, and he reported that palming and visualizing could calm even his worst moods.

He commented to me once that as he relaxed into palming, he was aware of strong tension in his neck and shoulders. I suggested that some good massages would loosen things up and support his eyesight as well. He began to go for weekly massages, and soon, his astigmatic condition was resolved and his eyesight continued to improve slowly.

Then in late summer, Alex decided he wanted to "trim up" and lose a few pounds, and so he took up running in the mornings. After running, he would palm for a long time before getting ready for work. He really loved this routine and I could see that he was feeling better about himself, generally.

I will never forget the final appointment I had with Alex, early that fall. He greeted me with a full, warm smile and a hug when I opened the door, and he sat down excitedly.

"I palmed my eyes for a long time the other night just before going to bed," he told me. "I'd had a terrible day and was thinking about another horrible, damn cold winter ahead. I had that feeling creeping up inside me; that feeling of hating everybody and everything ... but then, I started to palm and imagine the sun, and I was back in Greece again, and I'm so used to going there in my imagination, that I was soon feeling great and starting to get sleepy. I crawled into bed and went right to sleep. And then, at about 2:00 am I sat straight up in bed and said, out loud, 'I'm leaving Canada. I will not live here anymore. This is my decision, alone, and I'm going home!' I called in sick at work and that day I wrote my resignation. I called the consulate, told my parents and my girlfriend — of course, I'd like her to come with me, and she's thinking that part over — but whatever, I'll be back in Greece in three weeks!"

His eyes were full of tears, as were mine, and we shared another hug. Alex was really seeing again, in a profound and powerful way.

We said goodbye over the telephone a couple of weeks later and I wished him well on his new journey. His parents had been unexpectedly open to his plan, and they had promised to visit him in Greece within the next year. His girlfriend was still thinking about what to do, but was supportive of Alex's decision, because she could see how necessary this step was for him.

Alex thanked me for our work together and promised to keep up his vision practices. He said that he expected more and more clarity once he arrived in his home country. "You know, I feel so excited and positive about my life now, there is no more room for frustration or anger. Everything's just looking so good and is so clear to me now."

Indeed!

* * *

Having had that horrible experience on the airplane at age nine, Alex became terribly afraid of the future and of change, and that fear had become a part of who he was.

Alex justified keeping things "status quo" but actually, fear was so locked into his visual system that in my view, he had almost no choice. Once we had done the work of "unlocking" those chronically tensed eye muscles and a completely stressed visual system, circulation and energy began to flow again much more dynamically, and then things could change for him and be more to his liking.

He could literally see what was ahead, and make a fearless plan for his own future; a profound, life-changing plan.

* * *

Angelo's Story

Angelo was a man who attended my "Eight Weeks to Better Vision" course. He was a few minutes early for every class, had always completed all of his practices and the reading I had assigned, and was eager to begin each week.

Angelo also had the best vision of anyone there - 20/20 or better, and didn't wear glasses! Several of the students asked him early on why he was there. His response was interesting and very inspirational as well: "I want to see even better than I see now and just find out how far I can take this ... the whole subject fascinates me and I'm here to learn all that I can."

Angelo was a huge asset to our class, keeping it lively and more imaginative than it would have been without him. Everybody loved him and the contribution he made.

When our "Eight Weeks" was complete, we celebrated with a little party at one of the student's houses. We had come to know each other very well and there was a special cohesiveness in our group.

Towards the end of the evening, when everyone was finishing desserts and sipping tea, Angelo told us the rest of his story. Even I wasn't prepared for what we heard.

When Angelo was a young child in Tuscany, his mother was a struggling single mom, and Angelo was the eldest of four children who had been abandoned by their father. He was a great help to his mother through this time, and they were very close.

Angelo knew that his mother was "special" — apparently she could see angels hovering around people, she had premonitions about the future, and could sense when someone was about to make their transition to spirit, and she could often "read" people's thoughts. Many people in the village would seek out his mother when they needed advice.

This is where the story began to get really interesting … Angelo told us that in the summertime, he and his mother used to climb up onto the roof of their little house and "look for miles". He said his mother gently taught him the technique she used to "zoom over" to the next village (which was visible in the far distance), go onto the streets and look in the shop windows, and see who was there and what was happening. Angelo told us that he picked this skill up easily and he loved to sit with his mother and "zoom" around to the villages to see what was happening.

One time Angelo was actually visiting the neighbouring town with his mother and they saw his uncle there. Angelo innocently mentioned that he had seen him the day before from his rooftop, and saw him buying feed for his animals in the Farm Supply Shop. Angelo's uncle was very shocked, demanding to know how Angelo could do such a thing. His mother calmed his uncle with a white lie, and later explained to Angelo that he must never discuss what he'd "zoomed in on" because people didn't want to hear such things.

Young Angelo never discussed this ability again, but he secretly enjoyed using it to snoop around the different areas he could spy from his own rooftop. Angelo retained the ability to see in this profound way, he told us, all through his teen years until he was 19 years old. Suddenly that summer, his mother was killed by a drunk driver as she was walking along a dirt road, headed for home.

From the moment he heard the shocking news of his mother's death, Angelo could not "look for miles" anymore. His grief at losing his mother, and then being left to care for his younger siblings, was a big burden to bear ... but the children survived, and now Angelo was a man of 38, sitting with us and telling this fascinating story.

He said, "I've tried to 'look for miles' many times since — I've even returned to my home village recently and tried to 'zoom' there, but I just can't seem to do the same thing — whatever it was — with my eyes. I think it's partly because I've been taught that no one can see like that, but when I was with my mother, I knew that anyone actually could, if they were in that "space" I was in, when I looked. I was hoping that taking this course would tweak something, and I'd remember how it felt to see in that way. I believe that is the key; to go into that feeling, and then it just happens, and it feels completely natural, but it's awesome at the same time."

Since meeting Angelo, one of my clients told me that when he was in Nepal, he met and lived with sheepherders who could look many miles into the distance to spot and count every one of their sheep with their naked eyes. It seemed that they found missing sheep using this same "look for miles" technique. My client's belief was that they could do it because their fathers and grandfathers counted their sheep in this way, and "It never occurred to them that they couldn't." His repeated questions asking the sheepherders how they could see that far always evoked the same answer; "We just look out there and we see".

The extreme opposite to this kind of seeing would be the Chinese "rice writer" I met sitting outside of Granville Island Market in Vancouver, one sunny morning in July. She was a small lady, perched on a stool, writing people's names in beautiful calligraphy, on a single grain of rice. Some people requested their favourite quotes or love notes to others and the price went up according to how many characters she crafted onto the rice.

I was completely fascinated and waited my turn to have my name and a special quote written. She handed me a magnifier and showed me the words, then dropped the piece of rice into a tiny vial attached to a chain to hang around my neck.

By this time, I couldn't contain my excitement. I imagined this lady to be about 50 years old, but with incredible close focus; better than even very young children. I assaulted her with questions:

- How did she learn to see like this?

- Did she do something regularly to maintain this amazing close focus and to prevent eye strain?

- Did she go to school somewhere to learn this skill?

... and I had many more questions, but her response was short and simple:

"My whole family are rice-writers. I can see the rice because I need to see it, to do my work. This is the way I make my living. My father showed me how to do this, and he could write on rice until he was a very old man in his 80's. It's just what we do."

I asked her about her distance vision and she looked up towards the market entrance, about 20 feet away. She laughed and said, "I can't see anything over there. I don't need to."

These examples of amazing eyesight — young Angelo and his mother, the sheepherders, and the lady who writes on rice, all have one thing in common; they believed they could do this absolutely. My feeling is that when they were seeing in these various amazing ways, their eyes were relaxed, because they expected to see easily. Of course, there is so much more to know here about these people and how they did what they did. They all have one thing in common, however.

They were taught by the example of their elders ...

CONCLUSION

Young children everywhere today see glasses on about half of the people they look at. Their parents wear glasses, teachers wear them, and coaches and mentors of all kinds wear glasses in order to see clearly. We are not talking about anything unusual here. People are wearing glasses commonly in order to read and/or to see across the room. It has become "normal" and "normally" those lenses get stronger and stronger as life goes on.

But natural? I think not. We were meant to see naturally, with our own eyes working well and our visual system responding to every nuance of light and shadow, with all the clarity required available to us, for life.

It is definitely possible to reduce our dependence on those glasses, at any stage of life, clear up our vision and our perceptions, and look into the eyes of our babies and children without any barriers ... with love and energy and health, looking right back at us!

I'll finish as I began, with a quote from Gandhi:

"First they ignore you, then they laugh at you, then they fight you, then you win."

Certainly the ideas of William Bates and those who followed his lead have been ignored or mocked in some circles for many years. I hope I have demonstrated in this writing that Natural Vision Improvement stands as a simple and harmless alternative to the mainstream school of thought on vision.

It is my sincere belief that if we are willing to entertain the possibility that healing is something that our eyes can and will do, given the chance — naturally, and without risk - we have much to gain.

*If we can then begin to be more respectful of our eyes, **be easy on them**, treat them more gently and soothingly, and with understanding of their needs, we all stand to win.*

Joy Thompson
www.seeclearlynaturally.com
www.canadianvisioneducators.com

ABOUT THE AUTHOR

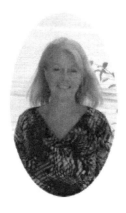

Joy Thompson has been working in the field of Natural Vision Education for eighteen years, since first improving her own eyesight in 1996. She is passionate about helping people to see better, feel better, and live healthier lives through improving the health of their eyes and the clarity of their seeing. Joy offers individual consultations, in person or long-distance, and leads workshops, seminars and retreats on Natural Vision Improvement.

www.seeclearlynaturally.com